In Pursuit of Garlic

IN PURSUIT OF

GARLIC

AN INTIMATE LOOK AT THE DIVINELY ODOROUS BULB

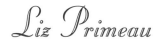

Liz Primeau

GREYSTONE BOOKS

D&M PUBLISHERS INC.

Vancouver/Toronto/Berkeley

Greystone Books
An imprint of D&M Publishers Inc.
2323 Quebec Street, Suite 201
Vancouver BC Canada V5T 4S7
www.greystonebooks.com

Cataloguing data available from Library and Archives Canada
ISBN 978-1-55365-601-2 (pbk.)
ISBN 978-1-55365-602-9 (ebook)

Editing by Nancy Flight
Cover and text design by Heather Pringle
Cover photograph by Julie Mcinnes/Getty Images
Illustration by Liz Primeau
Printed and bound in Canada by Friesens
Text printed on acid-free, 30% post-consumer paper
Distributed in the U.S. by Publishers Group West

We gratefully acknowledge the financial support of the Canada Council
for the Arts, the British Columbia Arts Council, the Province of British Columbia
through the Book Publishing Tax Credit, and the Government of Canada
through the Canada Book Fund for our publishing activities.

·Contents·

1

A DIVINE STINK

Garlic in History, Lore, Medicine, and More

The bulb, an oriental palace
shrouded in gray and lavender paper,
splits open into a heap
of wedge-shaped packets . . .

DAVID YOUNG, *"Chopping Garlic"*

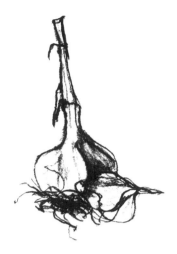

My *garlic bulb,* freed from the earth by my trusty trowel, is a moon more than a palace, a pearly orb with smears of dirt making a miniature Sea of Tranquility on its newborn skin. It's not as round as a moon, but it is undulating and sensual, with papery curves that hide Dracula's-fang cloves, their flavor so pungent that if I bite into one right away, it will sear my tongue and burn all the way down my throat.

But I won't do that. Garlic needs to mature and ripen to develop its best flavor, unlike carrots or parsnips or potatoes, which are at their crisp and sweetest best soon after they're pulled from the ground. Garlic is an opposite sort of root vegetable, whose taste improves with some age, becoming deeper and more layered.

I've cooked and savored this divinely odorous bulb, botanically known as *Allium sativum,* for many more years than I've grown it, but growing it has made me respect it. It's one tough little dude, a survivor with a history as long as the potato, and like the potato it's generally taken for granted. It's seen the rise and fall of civilizations and cultures and has made an appearance in the life of almost everyone who's ever lived. For about ten thousand years garlic has been many things: in Neolithic times it was a dependable food that could be kept fresh and edible in a cool cave for months. It's been a flavoring, a giver of strength, a healer, and a preventer of disease, and today it's being seriously studied for its medicinal value.

It shows up in literature, poetry, art, and architecture—early in the twentieth century Spanish architect Antoni Gaudí built a stylized garlic dome over an air vent on Barcelona's Casa Batlló, perhaps his take on the more familiar onion dome of Spain's Moorish history. Clay replicas of garlic or the real thing were buried with pharaohs and ancient kings to nourish and keep them safe from evil spirits as they passed into the great beyond. Images of garlic sometimes show up on hamsas, the hand-shaped amulets that protect against evil in the Middle East and North Africa. Garlic has appeared in paintings—two examples are Diego Velásquez's *A Young Woman Crushing Garlic* and Vincent Van Gogh's *Still Life with Bloaters and Garlic*—and references to garlic abound in literature. Shakespeare often alluded to it, usually disparagingly, in his plays; Cervantes, in *Don Quixote de la Mancha*, was critical of the smell of garlic on Dulcinea's breath; and one of Guy de Maupassant's characters in "The Rondoli Sisters" is downright disgusted by people who "carry about them the sickening smell of garlic." But in "Mandalay,"

Rudyard Kipling speaks lyrically of garlic: "You won't 'eed nothin' else / But them spicy garlic smells, / An' the sunshine an' the palm-trees and the tinkly temple-bells; / on the road to Mandalay…"

Garlic has also been used as currency. If I'd been an Egyptian four thousand years ago with a sackful of garlic bulbs to barter, I could have bought a healthy slave to help me with my garden. That sounds like a better deal than paying the neighborhood teenagers twelve bucks an hour to pull weeds and prune the hedge. Garlic had intrinsic value, too: if I'd been a stonemason working on a pyramid a millennium before that, I'd have been issued garlic every day to keep me strong and disease free. A record of labor costs inscribed on the Great Pyramid of Cheops showed that sixteen thousand talents of silver was spent during one bookkeeping period to feed garlic, onions, and radishes to the thousands of pyramid builders. A talent was an ancient unit of mass, the amount of water that would fill an amphora, and it was also used to measure precious metals. It's impossible to compare ancient and modern measurements or monetary values, but if one Egyptian talent was equivalent to 80 Roman libra, or about 57 pounds (26 kilograms), as Pliny said a couple of millennia later, these three humble vegetables were worth a lot indeed.

But more than painting or writing about garlic, or buying slaves with it, humans have always liked to eat garlic, whether it was considered good for your health or not. The Mesopotamians, a civilized people who lived in what is now mainly Iraq four thousand years ago, enjoyed garlic with abandon. Forty recipes inscribed on three clay tablets from about 1900 BC (translated from the cuneiform in the 1980s by French scholar Jean Bottéro and now part of Yale University's Babylonian Collection) use garlic and leeks liberally. The favorite technique was to mash and squeeze them through a cloth so that the juices were released into a pot of, say, mutton stew with beets and cumin. Garlic's green tops didn't go to waste either—they were marinated in vinegar and used to garnish the bowl.

Dear actors, eat no onions or garlic, for we are to utter sweet breath.

BOTTOM in *A Midsummer Night's Dream*

AS THE centuries rolled by, garlic's reputation as a health benefit didn't waver. Roman soldiers of the first centuries AD exuded clouds of garlic as they marched through Britannia and all the other countries they conquered, for they were issued several cloves of garlic a day to keep them strong and resistant to disease. Sailors plying the oceans reeked of garlic for the same reason. This belief in garlic's value as preventive medicine lives on, possibly for good reason. At the first sign of a cold or a touch of grippe my eighty-something father-in-law chows down on a clove of garlic to keep the germs at bay. He swears it works, and he's not the only person in the world who believes that a fresh clove, a few drops of garlic oil, or a homeopathic capsule will fend off disease, cure a touch of catarrh or treat a toothache.

And we all know that garlic keeps us safe from vampires, those blood-sucking beings who terrorized the Balkans and other parts of the world for centuries before becoming a household word with the publication of Bram Stoker's *Dracula* in 1897. Professor

Van Helsing crushed garlic flowers on the windowsills and doors of Lucy's room to keep the beast away, although judging by Francis Ford Coppola's 1992 movie version Lucy rather liked having him drop by at night.

. . . .

• BELIZE LOVE POTION •

Mix one clove of garlic, crushed, with a few leaves of rue plucked from your herb garden, a couple of hairs stolen from your lover's head, and a few threads from his or her underwear. Soak overnight in a generous shot of alcohol and strain. Offer to the object of your desire and take a sip yourself for good measure.

. . . .

Garlic has also come highly recommended as an aphrodisiac. In the first century AD Pliny the Elder wrote that to increase desire, garlic should be "pounded with coriander and taken with neat wine." In the Talmud, Ezra, a priest-scribe in about 450 BC, decreed that Hebrew husbands just returned to Israel from exile in Babylon should eat garlic on Shabbat to help them fulfill their marital duties and repopulate their homeland.

BUT DESIRE isn't always desirable. Pliny also advised that garlic should be eaten during festivals of abstinence because its powerful aroma discouraged sexual activity. Celibates of every belief generally abstain from garlic for fear it will stimulate prohibited passions. In India, visitors with garlic breath are unwelcome in many places of pilgrimage and in some mosques and temples; yet garlic is an important ingredient in Indian cooking and has always been integral to Ayurvedic medicine.

Ah yes, there's always been a hint of ambivalence when it comes to garlic. A fourth-century Buddhist medical treatise written in Sanskrit on birch bark (the Bower Manuscript, so named for the Indian army lieutenant who found it in the nineteenth century) waxed poetic about the garlic plant "with leaves dark blue like sapphires and bulbs white like jasmine, crystal, the white lotus, moonrays, or the conch shell," but the same manuscript also says that garlic sprang from the blood of a beheaded asura, a powerful being who was caught in the act of making off with the elixir of immortality. (A similar story with a Christian basis says garlic sprang from the footprint of Satan as he fled the Garden of Eden.) Even those garlic-loving Mesopotamians weren't allowed to eat it on the first three days of the year, when favors were being asked of the gods. You never know when a bad smell is going to make a god mad.

Garlic should be eaten in moderation
lest the blood of a man overheats.
HILDEGARD VON BINGEN, twelfth-century abbess and physician

MODERN GARLIC grows in two main types: hardneck (*Allium sativum* var. *ophioscorodon*), which grows a scape, or flower stalk, and softneck (*A. sativum* var. *sativum*), which doesn't. Under the two main groups, ten subgroups have been identified (they're listed in "A Garlic Primer," at the end of this book), though these subgroups keep changing as scientists conduct more research into garlic's genetics.

Hardneck garlic doesn't produce much in the way of flowers anymore, because procreation in this way has been bred out. It thrives in northerly climates with cold winters and is seldom, if ever, grown for large commercial purposes. Softneck garlic, which basks in milder climates, evolved from the original hardneck variety in the Mediterranean, where it was taken by adventurers and explorers in ancient times.

Garlic's lineage has been notoriously difficult to pin down, however. Even someone as acclaimed as Carolus Linnaeus—the mid-eighteenth-century Swedish botanist who studied and classified thousands of plants, listing their places of origin and giving them botanical names—said Sicily was its home. A century later another botanist, the Scotsman George Don, said Linnaeus might be right about the birthplace of softneck garlic but that hardneck garlic came from Greece or Crete. Softneck garlic had simply done what plants often do when they migrate to another country—it had adapted to a warmer climate and, as we shall see, began to reproduce essentially through its underground cloves, not via seeds. Did that make it a different species?

In 1875 Eduard Regel, a German botanist who was director of the Imperial Botanical Garden in St. Petersburg, Russia, said that the whole *Allium* genus—softneck and hardneck garlic, onions, leeks, shallots, and the ornamental alliums we grow in perennial borders—originated in Central Asia with the wild *Allium longicuspis*. His findings were accepted as the real thing for about a hundred years, partly because research into the family origins

of garlic wasn't big on everybody's list but also because the wild
A. *longicuspis* was found to be genetically identical to A. *sativum*,
our cultivated garlic (of both types).

Then, in 2008, a group of researchers led by Philipp Simon
in the Department of Horticulture at the University of Wisconsin
released DNA studies that suggest neither A. *longicuspis* nor
A. *tuncelianum*—another parental suspect—could be the ancestor.
Even today's botanists and scientists, who have studied garlic
with more advanced techniques than Regel's contemporaries
could have called upon, can't precisely date garlic's age or its
exact origins. They do agree, however, that hardneck garlic is
one ancient plant; it goes back at least ten thousand years to a
giant crescent of wild plants that grew through the mountainous
regions of Central Asia from Turkistan and the Celestial
Mountains into northern Iran.

For a common vegetable, garlic has a very mysterious ancestry.
But then how much do we know about the lineage of carrots or
any of the other vegetables we eat every day?

I must tell thee, Sancho, that when I
approached Dulcinea she gave me a whiff of raw garlic that
made my head reel and poisoned my very heart.

DON QUIXOTE

NO MATTER who *Allium sativum's* parents were, they had
strong survival instincts. The plants used their strong, stinging
sulfur compounds, which are released and combined when garlic is crushed or bitten (and which make it taste so good and are

credited with its medicinal qualities), to protect themselves from predators, parasites, and diseases. Yet the faintly pleasant aroma of the flowers attracted pollinators. Ancient garlic plants grew easily where many other plants couldn't survive—in rocky valleys, riverbeds, and gullies—and had strong roots that searched deeply for moisture and nutrients. The leaves were narrow and flat so the plants could withstand the heavy, quick frosts of Central Asia, and the plants learned to go dormant and live underground during the extreme heat and dryness of summer. They resumed growth quickly after a period of cold (called vernalization). When conditions above ground were inhospitable, the bulb established a root system that pulled the plant deeper into the ground with each passing season and thus ensured that it stayed anchored in the soil. Today's garlic has shallower roots, because the bulbs are harvested each year for human consumption and don't have an opportunity to dig deeper.

As insurance, ancient hardneck garlic had two means of procreation: the underground bulb, which had many cloves that produced new plants the next season, and the flowering stalk, or scape, which had an umbel at the end. Inside the umbel grew an intricate arrangement of tiny flowers and bulbils, which looked like miniature garlic cloves. When the umbels opened and the bulbils ripened, they dropped off and were carried by wind or water to a new place, where they'd take root and after several years develop into large, multicloved bulbs. The flowers in the umbel were fertilized in nature's tried-and-true method, by the birds and the bees, and after a few years' growth they too produced plants with strong, large bulbs.

• PLANTS FOR GOOD AND EVIL •

Until a couple of centuries ago plants were assumed to be possessed by gods or devils, as manifested by their smell or the shape of the root, bloom, or calyx. Mandrake root's resemblance to a male human form gave it many powers: it helped barren women conceive and men's passions to rise; it could also bring on madness, sleep, or death. Ginseng root shares a similar shape and was believed by the Chinese to contain the life-giving powers of the earth and thus to rejuvenate the old and sick. Garlic's smell and its shape affected its powers: even though it also grew in the earth, its aroma associated it with the evil underworld; its resemblance to a human head made it unacceptable to some vegetarians. Because they were black, urd beans and ancient fava beans were associated with death and were banned in some countries.

The banyan tree was sanctified because its roots grew downward from its limbs, bringing knowledge from the heavens; it and the pipal tree, another in the fig family, represented prosperity, safety, and fertility because it grew to be very old, with a massive trunk and spreading, protective branches.

Before too many millennia passed, garlic's distinctive qualities, especially its intriguing taste, were discovered by the people of the Neolithic period. It stored well and so provided necessary food and energy for the winter. Humans began to domesticate it. Explorers and travelers—including Marco Polo—journeying along the Silk Road of Central Asia were introduced to garlic;

they packed it in their caravans and took it with them as they moved around the ever-widening world—to North Africa, China, southern Asia, and the Mediterranean, where it was intensely cultivated and diversified and eventually, it is theorized, morphed into softneck garlic.

BUT GARLIC became famous among these cosmopolitan travelers as more than a food and a flavoring; it was also said to give men stamina and strength. It became prized for its reputed magical powers in repelling devils and dangerous stinging insects and in curing disease. Garlic became the trendy food of the age. The daughter of Mesopotamia's King Su-Su'en loved garlic so much that she took a whole trunkful with her on a trip to the kingdom of Ansan at the end of the third millennium BC. It was a huge crop in Egypt as well.

But popularity may have cost garlic its sex life. Gradually, over thousands and thousands of years, its birds-and-bees method of procreating has nearly disappeared. Garlic was a desirable crop and farmers were smart: they knew they could harvest better bulbs the following summer if they planted the cloves of especially desirable plants—those with stronger disease resistance, larger cloves, better taste, and greater storage capability. These bulbs were often produced by plants with weaker scapes and flower production (since the energies of those plants went into the bulb, not the flower), and as the centuries passed and plants with flowers were deselected, or flower scapes were deliberately removed to allow the growth of larger bulbs, garlic largely lost the ability to flower and set seed. Some flowers appear in today's hardneck garlic, but they've become impotent.

Poor garlic: no birds, no bees, no sex life.

But despite its centuries of evolution, our humble little friend is being reborn and is becoming the trendy food of the twenty-first century. It's undergoing a renaissance in the kitchen, the garden, and the medical laboratory. It's identified as one of the foods that provide that indefinable umami flavor, now widely accepted as the fifth taste, after sweet, salty, bitter, and sour. A high-priced fermented garlic with a pristine exterior and sweet, chewy black cloves has made its way into the best gourmet food shops, to be used on pastas, in salsas, with seafood—any way you can dream up. In the garden, growers are trying out dozens of new garlic varieties in varying shades and stripes of purple, red, white, and brown. There's even a pink one. The new cultivars don't taste like "just garlic" either—nuances abound from hot to mild, nutty to sort of sweet, though it's hard to describe garlic as sweet, because its strong essential flavor is always present. In late summer garlic lovers flock to fairs all over the continent offering the new varieties for sale, as well as lectures on raising and storing garlic and talks on its value for health.

There's a simple, though offbeat, explanation for all this interest: the falling of the Berlin Wall. "When it came down in '89, scientists were allowed into Russia and brought back literally hundreds of unnamed garlic varieties to North America for study," says Paul Pospisil, who owns Beaver Pond Estates in Maberly, Ontario, and is the largest trial grower of organic garlic in Canada, evaluating strains from all garlic groups for their performance on many levels before they're selected for further propagation. He's also the editor of the *Garlic News*, a publication much loved by garlic aficionados. "A large number of these Russian varieties have become the basis of the many new cultivars we see now," Pospisil continues.

Scientists' interest goes far beyond developing new garlic varieties, however, and their experimental work is bringing new respect to garlic's medicinal qualities. "Every university I know of is doing some kind of research into garlic," says Pospisil. "They're looking into its history and studying its taxonomy, of course, but most of all they're interested in its medicinal aspects."

With its selenium, germanium, allicin too
It can fight all kinds of disease
So if you've got arthritis, TB, or the flu
Just say, "Peel me a garlic clove please!"
RUTHIE GORTON, *"The Garlic Song,"* from the documentary
Garlic Is as Good as Ten Mothers, by LES BLANK

FOR AS long as people have been writing things down, garlic has been considered a healer of a long list of ailments, even as its culinary popularity waxed and waned. In 3000 BC the Babylonians used it to treat many ailments, including intestinal worms; so did the ancient Chinese—the *Chiu Huang Pen-ts'ao,* an important book of medicine from the Ming Dynasty, recommends garlic as a treatment for parasites, ringworm, and dysentery; a poultice for infections; an insect repellent; an expectorant; and a diuretic. In Ayurvedic medicine, Hindus considered garlic a general tonic and a digestive, and crushed and sweetened it with honey to relieve coughs and mucus, fevers, swellings, and worms. Sanskrit texts describe garlic as a remedy for skin and abdominal diseases, rheumatism, and hemorrhoids.

• GARLIC, THE WONDER DRUG •

In *Historia Naturalis,* Pliny the Elder wrote that garlic had powerful curative properties. "It's believed useful for making a number of medicaments, especially in the country," he wrote, suggesting that it was used more by rural folk than by city types.

· Pounded with vinegar and water, it was a gargle for "boils in the throat."

· Roasted and pounded with oil, it healed insect bites and bruises.

· Boiled with milk, it stopped catarrh.

· Roasted in live ashes, crushed, and taken with honey, garlic treated serious disease with "spitting of blood or pus."

· Mixed with fat, it cured tumors.

Pliny wasn't the only man of repute to consider garlic a cure-all. Several centuries earlier the Greek physician Diocles of Carystus prescribed it boiled as a cure for madness. Praxagoras blended it with wine to treat jaundice or mixed it with oil and a thick stew of grains for "iliac passion," a serious condition in which the bowel stops moving.

GARLIC WAS a wonder drug in ancient Rome and Greece, the kind of snake oil that charlatans might have peddled at carnivals in the early 1900s, recommended for baldness, cancer, and pale skin. Dioscorides, a discriminating Greek physician who served the Roman emperor Nero, warned that although garlic expelled flatulence, it could disturb the belly and cause thirst or boils on the skin if applied too heavily. But Dioscorides wasn't completely negative. He considered garlic valuable for many ailments. "It draws away the urine," he wrote in *De Materia Medica*, his five-volume study of the properties and preparation of contemporary drugs. He highly recommended garlic as an antidote for many poisons, to treat intestinal parasites, to protect against diarrhea caused by "injurious waters," to kill lice and nits, and to treat toothaches.

Perhaps more prophetically, given today's continuing research into the use of garlic to lower blood pressure and get rid of serum cholesterol, Dioscorides said garlic cleaned out the arteries and "opened the mouths of veins."

Or was it Pliny who said that? It's hard to know for sure, for both recommended garlic for similar ailments, and they were contemporaries. (Pliny died in AD 79, Dioscorides in AD 90.) Pliny's book was quoted for centuries, and Dioscorides's *De Materia Medica* became the main pharmacological work in Europe and the Middle East until the 1600s.

Garlic continued as a popular remedy for whatever ailed you during medieval times and the Renaissance. But by the twentieth century its good reputation had plummeted, despite the work of Louis Pasteur, who in the nineteenth century had recognized the antibacterial effect of garlic juice. Albert Schweitzer used garlic to treat amoebic dysentery in Africa in the early 1900s, but remedies based on superstition and old wives' tales were losing favor. By the 1930s, some of the new wonder drugs were already being prescribed.

Garlic was considered important when there was nothing else around, however. Medical staff on the front lines in the First World War made poultices out of garlic to treat wounds, and it was used in the Second World War when the new sulfa drugs and penicillin were unavailable. And garlic was used extensively to treat tuberculosis in the first quarter of the twentieth century. It's easy to dismiss garlic as a folk remedy that's been more efficiently replaced by modern drugs, but here's something to consider: our ancestors came to similar conclusions about garlic's medicinal properties while living continents apart and without print or electronic media to instantly broadcast their findings to the world. Afflictions like worms and intestinal parasites, diarrhea and other gastrointestinal disorders, coughs, bronchitis and pneumonia, skin lesions, hemorrhoids, infections of the ears and teeth—all were treated with garlic in some form.

GARLIC CONTAINS a wealth of sulfur compounds, which are well-known antibacterial agents, but allicin, an oxygenated sulfur, is the central compound most closely associated with garlic's therapeutic benefits today. (Allicin is also what gives garlic its pungent taste.) Curiously, allicin doesn't exist in an uncut clove but is born almost instantly when garlic is crushed or cut and two of its elements, alliinase and alliin, are released and rush headlong into each other's arms. All cooks are aware of this chemical reaction when they chop or crush garlic because they can smell it, even if they don't know the reason behind it. But this reaction wasn't understood until 1944, when Chester Cavallito, a researcher at a chemical company in New York City, isolated the compound and named it allicin. He, too, found that allicin had significant antibacterial activity, in some cases almost as effective as penicillin's.

• A CONTROVERSIAL CURE •

In the early 1900s William C. Minchin of Kells Union Hospital in Ireland used a face mask with the nose portion soaked in garlic to treat tuberculosis. He also recommended that patients chew garlic or use it in a throat spray for tuberculosis of the larynx. In both treatments, he wrote in his book *A Study in Tubercle Virus, Polymorphism, and the Treatment of Tuberculosis and Lupus with Oleum Allii*, the inhaled fumes acted as a germicide and destroyed the tubercles. At the time the *British Medical Journal* wrote that his success was remarkable, even though many patients couldn't tolerate the treatment and so gave it up. In the same issue another writer dismissed the doctor's success and said the cures were the result of good nursing, proper food, exercise, fresh air, and plenty of sleep.

In the decades since Cavallito's findings, research into the medicinal value of garlic has stepped up, even though the garlic remedies we can buy are still homeopathic preparations and health supplements whose content and quality are largely unregulated—in North America, at any rate. But today garlic is being studied for its lowering of blood pressure and serum cholesterol (clearing the mouths of veins!), antifungal activity and antibacterial qualities, lowering of blood sugars, and anticancer effects, as well as for its value as a pesticide.

Resistance to antibiotics is growing, and garlic could become a welcome alternative. In his richly informative book, *Garlic and Other Alliums*, State University of New York at Albany chemist Eric Block describes petri-dish tests comparing the effects of dilutions of fresh garlic and the antibiotic ampicillin on an E. coli bacterium. Garlic may not have performed quite as well as the antibiotic, but it definitely inhibited the bacterium's growth. In another test, a garlic solution caused E. coli bacteria to lose their shape, cluster together, and leak some of their contents. In experiments with strains of yeast such as candida, garlic was more effective than the fungal agent nystatin.

There's much more in Block's book—and many others— to persuade you to eat more garlic. The oral bacterium *Porphyromonas gingivalis*, which causes gum infections and has been associated with inflammation around the heart and rheumatoid arthritis, is sensitive to garlic. In a five-week trial, thirty people using a mouthwash containing 2.5 percent garlic showed reduced bacteria counts, and—probably much to the dismay of their nearest and dearest, although the test results didn't specify whether the scent of the mouthwash lived beyond the trial—the effect lasted for a couple of weeks after they'd stopped using the rinse. Clinical studies in the past decade also show that garlic packs a punch against *Helicobacter pylori*, which causes chronic gastritis and duodenal and gastric ulcers.

AS FOR its antiparasitic activity, crushed garlic mixed with alcohol has been used for centuries to treat amoebic dysentery, as Dr. Schweitzer knew, as well as giardiasis, malaria, sandfly fever, and sleeping sickness. And the common treatment today for

• ANTIFUNGAL TOENAIL REMEDY •

"I am not a physician and would guess that what helps one does not help all," says Chester Aaron, author of *The Great Garlic Book, Garlic Kisses*, and *Garlic Is Life*, plus many novels. "But this little remedy has helped fifteen people who contacted me; two said it did not help. Fungal infections of finger and toenails occur frequently, especially among older people, and meds can be very expensive. This treatment was given to me by a friend."

1 or 2 cloves of garlic
1 shot of vodka
small square of cotton

Press the raw garlic into the vodka in a small bowl. Dip the cotton into the vodka-garlic mix, squeeze it out, then place it on the nail—or nails, if more than one is affected. Cut a finger from a rubber glove and pull it over the toe and the cotton and secure it with a rubber band. Do this at night before bed and remove it in the morning.

Repeat every night for a week to ten days. One person said treatment required two weeks but was successful.

African eye worm, which afflicts millions in Cameroon and elsewhere in West Africa and is caused by the nematode *Loa loa*, is a mixture of onion and garlic juice dripped into the eye. In the past twenty years, garlic compounds have also shown some success in vitro against common viruses such as the herpes strain. The solution had to be so strong, however, that if it were used on living flesh it would damage the healthy cells around the treatment area. Many contemporary reports claim that garlic in some form— even consumed as part of a daily diet—prevents or inhibits the growth of malignant tumors. A 2009 in-vitro study tested extracts of various vegetables on cells from pancreatic, lung, stomach, kidney, prostrate, breast, and brain cancers, and garlic came out on top as the strongest inhibitor of cancer cell production. Results may be different in real life, however. But an epidemiological study of people in China compared the incidence of stomach cancer in two communities, one where average consumption of garlic was 0.7 ounces (20 grams) a day, and a second in which people ate less than 0.04 ounces (1 gram) a day (assuming an average clove weighs 2.5 grams, that's eight cloves and about half a clove, respectively). The incidence of cancer in the first group, which ate the larger amount of garlic, was 8 percent of the rate in the other group.

Tabloids helped make garlic the top-selling
single-herb supplement in 2006, [but] since their pages
also feature Elvis sightings and UFO bases on Mount Everest,
the legitimacy of their reporting is suspect.
ERIC BLOCK, *Garlic and Other Alliums*

THERE ARE many conflicting opinions about garlic and cancer, but enough evidence of its ability to inhibit cell growth exists that studies are taking place to determine how and why it might be effective against malignancies. Does it alter the metabolism of carcinogenic cells in some way? Does it somehow suppress their growth? Or does it simply improve the efficacy of other drugs? Or does it do any of these things?

As for cardiovascular disease, it seems the jury will be out for some time. Despite Dioscorides's and Pliny's conclusions that garlic opens the mouths of veins, most recent studies don't support the claims—most made by the manufacturers of garlic supplements—that garlic reduces cholesterol. A Stanford University clinical trial that compared the use of fresh garlic with the use of garlic capsules and powdered garlic in 192 adults showed... nothing. An Asian review of adults treated with garlic for moderately elevated LDL cholesterol concluded: "Garlic... shows no beneficial effect on serum cholesterol."

But does garlic reduce blood clotting, known in scientific circles as platelet reduction? Popular literature advises people about to undergo surgery to avoid garlic because it might thin the blood. In-vitro studies say that's possible, but most clinical trials suggest otherwise.

Many trials have taken place in the past decade to test this hypothesis, using volunteers who either took supplements or ate raw or cooked garlic (cooked garlic contains little or no allicin) in snacks or lunches. No platelet reduction was recorded in either group. But an Egyptian study showed that people who took aspirin along with garlic showed more occult blood in their feces and more gastrointestinal bleeding than a group who took aspirin alone, suggesting that the combination reduces clotting more than either garlic or aspirin alone.

As for reducing blood pressure, some tests in the 1990s showed promising results, though they were primarily designed to measure blood lipids, not blood pressure. Two studies in the past decade showed that garlic reduced systolic pressure as well as commonly prescribed blood pressure drugs did. Then another study showed no significant results.

So you can see where this is going: there's no conclusive evidence that garlic successfully treats cardiovascular problems. You can pretty much believe what you want—or eat your clove of garlic a day mainly because you love the stuff and hope for the best. Garlic's antibacterial, antifungal, and antiparasitic value and its apparent ability to reduce elevated blood glucose— even its potential as a type of treatment for cancer—have more promise.

As Block says in his book, garlic displays remarkable in-vitro activity in many areas, and much of this activity is borne out in in-vivo studies with rats and other lab animals. But more study and more human trials are needed before garlic's medicinal value can be established. Some substances in our bodies deactivate garlic compounds as soon as they enter our systems, so that many elements that show up in petri dishes are broken down in the body, making them less active as healing compounds. Block dreams of a day when garlic's healing compounds are packaged in little pills or some other kind of delivery system that will take them directly to the part of the body that requires treatment, bypassing metabolic degradation.

Maybe when that happens, garlic will become the newest miracle drug, not just the latest trendy food.

A PUNGENT LOVE AFFAIR

The Art of Eating Garlic

———————— ◦ ————————

Tomatoes and oregano make it Italian;
wine and tarragon make it French...
Soy sauce makes it Chinese; garlic makes it good.

ALICE MAY BROCK, baker of hash brownies;
owner of Alice's Restaurant;
author of *Alice's Restaurant Cookbook*

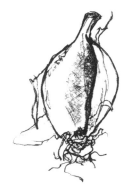

The night I discovered garlic, my thoughts were on anything but food. I was seventeen, madly in love as only a hormone-fueled teenager can be, with a gorgeous black-haired boy with dimples and white teeth. He'd borrowed his father's car for an evening drive-about, our euphemistic term for a quick tour of the city's streets and then a long park somewhere dark. These evenings were relatively innocent compared with what I hear about teenage sex lives today, but they were exciting and risky then, sometimes involving a roving and perhaps overzealous policeman who shone a flashlight into the car window. What if he took the license plate number and called Joe's father? Or, worse, my mother?

Never mind, the risk was worth it. This particular occasion was a hypnotic spring evening in early June trembling with promise. The soft air smelled deliriously of lilacs and wrapped around us like eiderdown. The sky was streaked with pastel clouds. But June days are long, and it was taking forever for the sun to go down. We'd driven down every street we cared to, and there was still too much daylight for parking.

"Well, how about we go for some spaghetti?" asked Joe, stopping the car in front of a tiny restaurant across from our favorite park. We'd passed it many times but had never gone in. A restaurant wasn't my idea of a comfortable place to be with a boyfriend, especially a restaurant that served spaghetti. Eating dinner with Joe's family was a test I'd managed to pass without choking on the roast beef, but I couldn't imagine slurping up a dish of slippery pasta in front of him. But he flashed his disarming dimply smile, and we got out of the car.

Peering through the small window in the door covered by an iron grille, we glimpsed dark booths and amber lights inside. The wooden door was heavy, and we both had to push hard to open it. We laughed when it gave and we nearly fell over the threshold. I took a deep breath and was stopped mid-inhale by the most gloriously pungent, tastebud-tingling aroma I had ever encountered. I forgot my eating anxieties instantly; even the anticipation of the main intent of the evening vaporized.

Stop and smell the garlic. That's all you have to do.
WILLIAM SHATNER

THE ROOM emanated a conglomerate of almost visible aromas— tomato, oregano, hot peppers, cheese—bound together with an indescribably rich, deep, almost skunky smell. It was garlic, of course, my first smell of the real thing. It's unfair to use the word *skunky* to describe a smell so deep, dark, and delicious, but skunk spray and garlic bulbs do have something in common: sulfur compounds. Once I heard someone describe skunk spray as a combination of rotten eggs, burnt rubber, and garlic, which I guess is fairly accurate, though I fear it casts aspersions on one of my favorite foods.

"*Mmmmmm*... what *do* I smell?" I asked the restaurant's black-vested waiter, a boy not much older than the two of us. He'd met us at the door, bowing slightly and whisking a large red napkin past his body in a theatrical gesture that invited us in.

"My dad's spaghetti and garlic meatballs," he said proudly. "The best this side of Sorrento, where we come from."

He beamed at us as he led the way through the dim, cozy room to a booth. The table was covered with a red-checked cloth, and in the center a Chianti bottle dripped candle wax. Squat shakers of grated cheese and dried hot peppers sat on each side. It was the kind of place I'd consider the ultimate cliché nowadays, but that night it seemed impossibly sophisticated.

"Do you want menus tonight?" the waiter asked, looking a bit anxious. We were the only people in the room.

"Um, okay," we said in unison. In the chrome and Formica establishments where we usually ordered toasted BLTs, the menu was either tucked behind the quarter-a-song jukebox on the wall or slapped on the table by the waitress. Here our waiter presented two leatherette-bound volumes with a flourish and then hovered over us, making me uncertain. There were too many unfamiliar things to choose from. And were we actually going to eat a meal?

"Any questions about our selections?" he asked, sounding a little rehearsed. "Everything is home cooked, in the Italian way, by my mom and dad. The spaghetti and meatballs are my dad's specialty, although there are some seafood items you might like, or perhaps some ravioli stuffed with veal?"

"I think I'll have the spaghetti and meatballs," I said. I wanted to taste that delicious smell, and I'd never eaten veal or even heard of ravioli.

With our identical orders written carefully on his pad, the waiter retreated to the kitchen and came back with a basket of toasty bread oozing butter and garlic. I bit into a piece, and it was heaven, the aroma at the doorway multiplied a thousand times into a taste that filled my mouth as well as my nostrils. After the first bite I didn't care about the butter sliding down my chin. I had a second slice, and then a third. When the basket was empty, the waiter looked very pleased and brought us another, followed by big flat bowls of spaghetti glistening with tomato sauce and topped with three meatballs the size of golf balls.

I didn't think I'd eat the whole thing, but I did, savoring each bite of soft, garlicky meatball and letting the spaghetti and slippery sauce roll around my mouth before I swallowed it. I slurped it, too—we both did, and it was a bonding moment between us, when we both managed to put aside our self-consciousness and simply eat with gusto, no matter what we looked like.

I'd never eaten such a heavenly meal. That evening was the first of many visits to "our" Italian restaurant, and Luca, the waiter, became almost a friend. He always greeted us with a wide smile and a basket of hot garlic bread. I thought he was psychic. How did he know we were coming? Did he have a basket ready every evening at seven in case we dropped by? We ate the same meal every time, too, partly in honor of that first evening, but mainly because we loved it so much. It was our tradition.

I've often wondered what became of that restaurant, whose name I can't remember, and of Luca and his beaming smile. The cozy, welcoming atmosphere and his dad's Promethean cooking had a big influence on me. It was a very long time ago, but that evening was a turning point in my life. It opened up a new world of taste and provided me with one of the keenest—and the garlickiest—gastronomic experiences of my life.

My eyes grew heavy and I began to sink into an odd,
sleepy euphoria. "Ah," said Robert. "She is feeling the garlic effect."
RUTH REICHL, *Comfort Me with Apples*

I DIDN'T realize that Luca and his family were going to have an influence on more than my budding sense of taste. They were a small part of the contingent of thousands of Italians and other Europeans who immigrated to North America—and particularly to Toronto, where I lived—right after the Second World War. They brought garlic with them, but they brought other influences too: they cried and they laughed more and harder than my Anglo-Saxon family did, they had bigger families that interacted more, and they went to church a lot, grew their own vegetables, and made their own sausages and wine. They almost always created their own communities and stayed within them, even though my grandma sniffed that "those new people" didn't know their place. She meant, of course, that their place was anywhere but our country, but since they were here they'd better learn not to upset the British status quo.

I loved Grandma, but she was a bit of a relic, if not an outright bigot. She was an immigrant herself—she'd come to Canada from Britain as a young mother with Grandpa and my father. Despite her wacky sense of humor and lively nature, she had a disapproving side and stood firmly on guard for staid British ways. Her new country never measured up to her old one, but whenever a few "vulgar foreigners" threatened our conservative British colony, she rose to its defense as if it were Buckingham Palace under attack. Not for anything or anyone would we relinquish our refined ways, especially not for those Johnny-come-latelies who were not original settlers. This was Britain's country.

Grandma didn't live to see the changes, but within a generation all of those foreigners—the Italians, the Portuguese, and the Greeks, and later Indians, Poles, Vietnamese, Chinese, and more—had started to reshape life and attitudes in many parts of the continent for the better, bringing an exciting mixture of cultures that has continued in the generations since.

None of this was obvious to me on those adolescent evenings when Joe and I ate spaghetti and meatballs in Luca's restaurant and gazed hungrily into each other's eyes. But when we were married and had our own apartment kitchen, I began to practice my newly discovered hobby: cooking. This was a new adventure with unseen boundaries. In the produce department of our local supermarket I found vegetables that Grandma had never seen, "exotic" ones like zucchini and eggplant. Even broccoli, which had been around for a few years but was generally disdained because of its cabbagelike taste, was gaining in popularity. Garlic was significantly absent. It never grew in my father's vegetable garden so I'd never laid eyes on it and I assumed it grew in the tropics, maybe on a tree. But garlic salt and garlic powder lurked on the spice shelves. I bought some of the powder but wasn't sure how to use it, so it languished in my kitchen cupboard until it yellowed and hardened and I threw it out, wondering if I was missing something.

Italian eateries were sprouting up all over, and spaghetti became a staple on the tables of Anglo-Saxons like me—spaghetti with meat sauce, not the big, soft meatballs that Luca's dad made. Even he morphed our favorite dish into spaghetti Bolognese, a North American version of a classic Italian recipe. Every restaurant served it, and every new cook and college student on a budget had his or her own version. The home versions were made with ground beef sautéed and then simmered with copious quantities of canned tomato sauce—and not much garlic or any other herb except for a pinch of dried basil. The authentic Bolognese recipe—named for Bologna, where it originated—is made with pancetta and beef, veal and/or pork (sometimes chopped, not ground), minced onion, carrot, celery, plenty of garlic, red wine, chicken stock, a bit of tomato paste, and a cup or so of milk to smooth and enrich the sauce. It's thick, more like a meat stew than a tomato sauce, and is usually served with tagliatelle, not spaghetti, although that's a niggly point. It's also great with polenta.

I'd never heard of tagliatelle when we went to Luca's restaurant, and I doubt that it was on the menu. Spaghetti was the pasta of the day, with lasagna a close second, prepared with the ever-present meat sauce layered with lots of mozzarella cheese. I didn't know that in Italy pasta was often served just with masses of chopped garlic, olive oil, and Parmesan cheese, the best way ever. It and many other variations, including an authentic Bolognese sauce, can be found in North American restaurants today because we've learned to love real Italian food and to adore garlic. People like Luca and his family got the changes rolling, and gradually the meat-and-potatoes dinner lost its place at the top of the North American meal plan, which began to include soupçons of garlic.

Unless very sparingly used,
the flavour is disagreeable to the English palate.

ISABELLA BEETON,

Beeton's Book of Household Management (1861)

BOTH MOM and Grandma, who lived with us, were good cooks, but our meals always followed the meat-and-potatoes plan and seldom had strong flavors—certainly never a hint of garlic. We rubbed thyme and sage on our pork chops, doused them with HP Sauce, and considered ourselves adventurous gourmands. When I look at the label on the bottle of HP Sauce stored in my fridge, I'm surprised to see garlic on the ingredients list. Who knew?

Garlic was never chopped into Grandma's steak and ale pie, and slivers of garlic were never inserted in Mom's roast beef. Funny, I'm just one step removed from that English heritage, but I can't imagine roast beef without a couple of cloves of garlic sliced and embedded in the succulent meat.

Mom and Grandma hadn't been introduced to the wonderful allure of garlic, but there was more to their avoidance of the odorous bulb than a lack of opportunity. They'd inherited the Anglo-Saxon prejudice against it. Even when I was a little girl I'd often heard Grandma speak disdainfully of "that man across the street, the one with garlic on his breath." It appeared he was more unworthy than the lurching fellow down the street, whose breath was often rank with beer. Their prejudice wasn't their fault, I suppose. For long stretches of history, from the Romans to the Renaissance and for most of the twentieth century, Anglo-Saxons scorned garlic as fit only for peasants. Garlic isn't used much by the Japanese, either, perhaps because Japan is geographically isolated and its food has traditionally been based on local products, yet it's an essential part of other Asian cuisines—Korean, Thai, Indonesian, and Chinese. Maybe the Japanese are like the English and have an aversion to foods considered attractive to peasant stock.

Long before the Romans invaded Britannia, their soldiers knew that garlic was good for more than keeping muscles strong. It also gave a pot of plain old turnips a boost. The soldiers passed their kitchen tricks along to Celtic cooks—sometimes men, sometimes women, for the Celts had a democratic society in which women were considered equal to men, owned property, chose their own husbands, and led battles, as Queen Boudicca did. And little by little, won over by the growing variety of other vegetables and fruits the invaders brought from their warmer Mediterranean country, the Celts learned to appreciate garlic.

The Romans introduced many foods to Britannia during the nearly four hundred years they occupied the country. They also built roads that lasted for centuries, founded cities like London and Manchester and York, created water and sewage systems, and established linear measurement. You might say they started

Britannia on the road to civilization. Their influence continues to this day (in Canada we started to phase out feet and inches in favor of metric measurement a couple of decades ago, but many of us still prefer the Roman way) and this includes their effect on the Celtic diet. The Celts were big on hunks of ox or cow speared right out of the pot with a knife, but the Romans introduced them to chicken; different kinds of game, including brown hare and pheasant; and a delicious escargot (*Helix pomatia*), called the Roman snail in Britain today. They brought herbs such as parsley, thyme, bay, and basil; fruits such as apples, mulberries, and cherries; and many vegetables, including cabbages, peas, and asparagus. And they brought garlic, as well as leeks, onions, and shallots—all members of the *Allium* genus. The leek was adopted so wholeheartedly that it later became the national emblem of Wales.

Putting aside the soldiers who stank of garlic, it's fair to say the Roman generals and bureaucrats were a pretty impressive lot. They were civilized and sophisticated, and they knew how to prepare food and eat it with ceremony. Soon the Celtic elite—for there was an elite in Britanny, made up of chieftains and tribe rulers, not to mention Druid priests—began to suffer from an ancient version of Stockholm syndrome, and within a generation or two they were emulating the ways of their invaders. They invited the Romans to fancy dinner parties, ordering fine foods and wines from around the empire to impress them. The two groups intermarried. The Celts took up the Roman practice of reclining on couches to dine and kept slaves to serve and mop up. One woman in Chester, England, was so won over by the Roman way of dining that she had a likeness of herself lounging in typical Roman fashion in her triclinium carved on her tombstone. Her guests might have been served nettle pie, roast duck in fancy sauces of dried damson plums or other fruits, swan simmered in seawater, and steamed custards of small fish. The upper classes ate dishes flavored with garum, a fermented fish sauce much like the Vietnamese nam pla we use today, and Asian spices such as ginger, pepper, cinnamon, and saffron.

But no garlic.

As far as the Roman aristocracy was concerned, garlic was fine for giving strength to those who needed it or for providing the peasants' humble food with more flavor, but they didn't touch the stuff themselves unless it was prescribed by the family physician for a poisonous bite of the shrewmouse or an attack of asthma. Among the upper classes garlic was considered a tonic and a medicine—it was used more than any other herb in the pharmaceuticals of Greek and Roman times.

Meanwhile, by the fifth century the Roman empire had come to its inevitable end and a dark age was casting its gloom over the world. Roman soldiers and their leaders left Britannia, and food became simply a necessity again. Garlic continued to grow around the abandoned garrisons and was harvested by the peasants and farmers descended from the Celts who'd learned its value in a pot of turnips, but in most of the country a bias against garlic as food took hold and lasted for centuries. Come to think of it, it lasted until my grandma's day.

It was the monks who kept both garlic and all of Europe alive during those impoverished days. The early Middle Ages was a good time to be a monk: at that time monks were probably the most economically advantaged people in the world. Their monasteries were both physical and spiritual sanctuaries, where good food (we can only assume some of it was cooked with garlic) and good health were encouraged. Good health included good medicine, and the monks had the time and the wherewithal to study and make many medicines from plants, including garlic.

OTHER NORTHERN Europeans weren't quite as snooty about garlic as the English. Poles, Russians, Germans, and Hungarians knew a good thing when they smelled it and adopted garlic as a flavoring, though not as wholeheartedly as people living around the Mediterranean. During the Renaissance, after fourteen-year-old Catherine de' Medici of Florence married France's equally young Henry II, in 1533, and brought her own chefs to France with her, the French grew to love garlic also. Those in the northern part of the country, however, always held themselves a little aloof from garlic's strong flavors and used it only in small quantities. Henry IV, who in 1600 took one of Catherine's cousins, Marie de' Medici (who was as influential as Catherine in culinary matters), as his second wife, was a devout garlic lover, maybe because a clove of garlic was rubbed on his lips when he was born to protect him from evil spirits. He regularly ate so much raw garlic it's said his breath could knock out an ox at ten paces.

With enough garlic, you could eat the New York Times.

MORLEY SAFER

EVENTUALLY I married the beautiful Joe and was embraced by his family. As third-generation descendants of Irish and English

• BARBECUE TIPS
FROM THE TWELFTH CENTURY •

England's upper class had at least one garlic lover in medieval times: Alexander Neckham, theologian, poet, grammarian, biblical scholar, gourmand, and accomplished cook, born in 1157, on the same night as Richard I. In fact, Alexander shared his mother's milk with Richard, since his mother was Richard's wet nurse. Because of his talents as a cook and a storyteller, Alexander was a popular host of dinner parties. He lived for several years in France and could offer cooking advice that would stand up among today's backyard barbecue chefs.

"A roast of pork is prepared diligently," he wrote, "[if it is] frequently basted, and laid on the grid just as the hot coals cease to smoke. Let condiments be avoided other than pure salt or a simple garlic sauce. It does not hurt to sprinkle a cut-up capon with pepper. [It will] be quite tender turned on a long spit, but it needs a strong garlic sauce, diluted with wine or verjuice."

immigrants, with a touch of French in the mix that shows up in the surname I still carry, my in-laws were almost as Anglo-Saxon as my family.

My mother-in-law loved to cook almost as much as she loved to say the rosary and go to Mass, though I'm sure cooking two and sometimes three squares a day for seven people was a

• KEEP YOUR POWDER DRY •

Garlic powder may not have the lively taste or health benefits of fresh garlic, but it can come in handy as a last-minute flavor fix in the kitchen. To maintain at least some of its goodness, commercially produced garlic powder is cut and dried at about 122°F (50°C) and no higher than 140°F (60°C), then crushed. It's at least twice as concentrated as fresh garlic, and the taste is a little different because of the sulfur compounds released during the cutting and drying. But the potential for some allicin production remains, and most dried powders contain more of the benefits of fresh garlic than do the blanched or acidified whole cloves sold in packages. Naturally, quality varies among products. Garlic powder has a long shelf life and maintains its qualities for three years or more if it's kept dry.

chore. She was a born cook, and she liked to try new recipes on her gleaming white stove, which I coveted. Instead of a regular cooking element on the rear left, it had a deep well with an extra-low heat setting for simmering stews and soups, something like a built-in slow cooker, a feature I never saw again. It was a good idea that should be resurrected. She used it to make one of her new specialties, "Eyetalian" spaghetti sauce, a version of a recipe she'd picked up from the Italian wife of a local butcher.

One day she taught me how to make it. "Chop the onion small and fry it first," she instructed, tying the strings of her big apron behind me. "Don't let it get too brown. Stir it around and let it sauté a bit."

She had a whole set of wooden spoons I thought were quaint and old-fashioned, though I admitted grudgingly to myself that they stayed cool even if you left them in the pot by mistake. Then she crumbled in the "pound of ground round" she'd bought from the butcher's wife, specially selected for her from very lean trimmings of bottom round steak. "Never add it in one lump," she said, "or that's the way it will stay." The meat was further broken up with vigorous fork action, which I had to watch before I was allowed to do it.

When the meat was browned and suitably separated, she gave me a big can of stewed tomatoes to open, pour in, and mush around in the pot. Then a can of tomato paste and pinches of dried basil and oregano. I stirred, and the greenish-black bits gave up their fragrance to the bubbling sauce. "And now," my mother-in-law announced dramatically, "here is the butcher's wife's little secret." And she produced a small cellophane packet of white powder. "Only a tiny bit of this now—we don't want to make it too strong and smell the house up."

IT WAS garlic powder. I took a sniff. It reminded me of that wonderful smell in Luca's restaurant, but not exactly. It was harsher, a bit like tin. The tiny pinch I stirred into the bubbling sauce was quickly swallowed up, and then a fuller, subtler aroma was released. Why hadn't I opened the package in my kitchen before it crystallized and turned yellow?

The cooking well was covered, the heat turned to the slowest simmer, and the sauce left all afternoon to cook down and thicken up. We consumed it steaming hot, over coils of thick spaghetti, with lashings of grated Parmesan shaken from a supermarket container.

I was grateful for the cooking lesson and took the recipe home in my head. I made it at least twice a month but added my own embellishments, because, like my mother-in-law, I liked to experiment. Over the years I used more and more garlic powder until the sauce did smell up the place, in a good way, of course. Then I introduced chopped celery and green peppers. Once I added pineapple chunks, a hideous mistake. I started adding a pinch of sugar if the tomatoes seemed too tart. A few times I snuck in a dash or three of hot pepper sauce, until the children— for by this time we had four, three eating adult food and one still on canned purées—complained that it was too "'picy."

My mother-in-law's sauce, formerly the butcher's wife's sauce, had become my sauce, and I took full credit for it if anyone commented favorably on its taste. I'm more honest now and can freely admit my mother-in-law was my inspiration. For years it was my only sauce, but then I learned a new method directly from another Italian woman: Anna, a handsome, big-boned woman who helped me clean the suburban house we'd settled into.

Anna saw me making my sauce one day and stopped to comment, though that was rather difficult since she didn't speak much English. But she got her point across with a torrent of Italian accompanied by many gestures toward my simmering sauce and a sweeping-away motion toward the opened cans of tomatoes and the bottles of garlic powder and herbs on my counter. *"Fresca, fresca,"* she said emphatically. Her meaning wasn't hard to ascertain. Her last gesture was a finger pointing to her chest, followed by a familiar thumb-and-forefinger circle at her mouth and a loud lip-smacking *mmm-wah!* Her show-and-tell was clearly meant to let me know she made a really, really good tomato sauce, better than I ever could with my bottled herbs and dried garlic and canned tomatoes.

On her next cleaning day Anna brought me a plastic tub of her sauce.

"*Mangia, mangia,*" she commanded, opening the tub and handing me a spoon. I complied—what else was I to do?—and even though the sauce was cool and not accompanied by a pasta partner, it made me close my eyes with pleasure. I was transported back to Luca's restaurant and the aroma and flavor of tomatoes melded with cheese and that rich undertone of garlic.

"Mmmm," I said, opening my eyes. Anna was waiting for my reaction and was clearly pleased. With a dramatic flair she'd obviously been born with, she set a plastic shopping bag on the counter and with a flourish withdrew a huge preserving jar of tomatoes, a wedge of Parmesan, a whole uprooted basil plant, a big yellow onion, and a huge bulb of garlic. Today we were going to cook, not clean.

Anna set to it. With authority she pulled the rolling pin and a big carving knife from a drawer, set the garlic bulb on my wooden breadboard, and with a quick, light whack of the rolling pin separated the bulb into papery cloves. Then she smashed the flat of the knife blade down on each clove, one after the other, instantly releasing that strong and wonderful smell of garlic. The skin was set aside and the smashed cloves were expertly minced, then the onion quickly peeled and chopped fine. Into a saucepan they both went—and I mean *the whole bulb of garlic*—with

· ·

• ANNA'S SAUCE •

Anna didn't use measurements when she made her ambrosial sauce, but I developed rule-of-thumb instructions so that I could pass a recipe along to people who asked. Instead of tomato purée I often use canned plum tomatoes—a 28-ounce can plus a 19-ounce can—puréed in my food processor. The taste and texture of the sauce varies slightly every time you make it—it depends on the thickness of the purée and the sweetness of the tomatoes.

1 medium	onion
1 whole bulb	garlic
2 tbsp	olive oil
two 25-ounce jars	tomato purée, about 6 cups
1 cup	freshly grated Parmesan cheese
½ cup	chopped fresh basil
	(use 1 tbsp or more to taste
	of dried basil if fresh is unavailable)
	salt and pepper to taste

Peel and chop onion into small dice. Separate the garlic bulb into cloves, peel them, and chop finely. In a large saucepan, heat the oil and sauté onion until it begins to color—don't brown. Add garlic and sauté just until it's fragrant.

Add tomato purée and bring to a gentle boil. Turn heat down, cover saucepan with a lid, leaving it partly open, and simmer gently for about 45 minutes, no longer than an hour. Cooking time depends on the thickness of the bottled purée; because they have more liquid, canned tomatoes need about an hour to thicken slightly. Add Parmesan and stir till it melts. Turn off heat and add basil, salt, and pepper. Allow sauce to sit for a day before using it for pasta al pomodoro: boil a pasta of your choice to just short of al dente; drain and return to the pot with a little of the pasta water and a dash of olive oil and a knob of butter. Cook until mixture thickens a bit, then fold in some of the tomato sauce—don't drown the pasta; the Italians never do! Garnish with lots of grated Parmesan and more chopped basil.

. . . .

a dash of olive oil, to sauté slowly and fill the kitchen with that irresistible aroma of two alliums cooking.

"Mmmmm," I said again. Anna grinned. She was enjoying this. She pulled my bottle of garlic powder from the spice shelf and tossed it into the garbage. I flinched. "No, no," she said firmly. *"Quello fresco,"* she insisted. I had to admit that her fresh garlic smelled better than my dried stuff. The preserving jar was opened and its contents went into the saucepan—a purée of red ripe tomatoes, not stewed or whole. *"Io li ho cresciuti e preservati,"* she said. What did she mean? I shrugged my shoulders and raised my eyebrows.

Anna made a digging motion and pantomimed putting a plant into the ground and patting the soil around it. *"Io li ho piantati e cresciuti da me stesso,"* she said, gesturing to my tomato bed at the back of the house. It was her body language that did it. The big jar was filled with tomatoes she had grown, just as I had grown mine, and had preserved herself, as I had not. I pointed to the basil and raised my eyebrows again. Anna nodded. She'd grown the basil herself, too. And the garlic? I pointed at the bits of skin on the cutting board. She nodded again. Even then I was a pretty serious gardener, but, except for the tomatoes in the sunny spot behind the house, I wasn't interested in growing vegetables or herbs, and I'd never known anyone who grew garlic. But she was Italian, and it was probably a native plant where she came from. Was it difficult to grow? Maybe I could try some myself sometime. But our language differences made it too difficult to ask Anna more, so I filed my thoughts away for the future.

Anna put the lid on the pot, leaving a crack open at one side, turned down the heat, and pointed to her watch. "Now we clean," she said in English.

About forty-five minutes later Anna gestured to me to return to the kitchen. She grated the cheese and added about a cup to the sauce, along with salt and pepper. She stripped the leaves off the basil plant and handed me a knife. Chopping the basil was to be my contribution. In went the little mound of green, and then Anna stirred the mixture until the cheese melted, turned off the heat, and let the pot sit on the warm element.

"*Mangiare domani,*" Anna said, tapping the rim of the pot and shaking her head. "*Non oggi.*" I understood instantly, as one cook to another. Let it sit for a day so that the flavors develop. Eat it tomorrow, not today.

WE DID eat it tomorrow, and we all had Roman-soldier breath the day after that. The sauce was delicious, rich yet light, with an exhilarating, fresh gardeny taste of tomatoes enriched with the deep flavors of the cheese and garlic. The kids gobbled it up. I decided the fresh taste was due as much to the relatively short simmering time as to the homegrown and home-preserved tomatoes it was made with. A rich tomato sauce that's been cooked down all afternoon has its place all right, such as spread on pizza, dabbed on green beans, or served sparingly with meatballs, but sometimes it can be heavy and tongue-burningly strong. The texture of Anna's sauce was finer than mine, too, with no lumpy pieces of tomato, because of the puréeing process. Until I eventually bought my own tomato mill, which grinds the raw fruit whole and then discards the skins and seeds—and is made in Italy, I might add—I replicated the texture by puréeing tomatoes in a blender or, once I acquired one, a food processor. But it was all the garlic that was the clincher, and I knew it. That round, full flavor, like the bass in a jazz quartet.

Eat it. Love it. The odds are high that garlic
will love you in return. Can you say that about thyme? About sage?
About arugula? About your child?

CHESTER AARON, *The Great Garlic Book*

FOR MANY years Anna's sauce replaced my mother-in-law's in its various Canadian-style versions as my new official pasta sauce. I adhered religiously to Anna's method and never added green peppers, celery, or other exotica. And I never altered its secret ingredients: an *entire bulb* of garlic—when I could get my hands on the real thing, that is (I'd rescued the bottle of dried stuff Anna unceremoniously threw into the garbage can and used it till it was gone, then bought another one and another one)—and the grated Parmesan, melted right into the mixture. Sometimes, I confess, I was reduced to using the supermarket shaker can. Back in the mid-sixties, it was difficult to buy whole wedges of fresh Parmesan, but as new Canadians kept arriving to lay the bricks or pour the foundations of the new houses in Toronto's burgeoning subdivisions or to open new restaurants, stores began to stock it. It was expensive—and it still is—but its full, nutty flavor and moist freshness is worth every penny.

As for garlic, it started to show up on some greengrocers' shelves, but it didn't look like the one Anna had brought to my kitchen. Hers had almost filled my palm, its shiny skin striped with purple. The all-white store-bought ones were piddlingly small and too often had green shoots in the center and rotten cloves that turned into gray powder inside their papery covering as soon as I tried to pull them off.

But after years of searching for good garlic, I got lucky.

Although we lived in a WASPy subdivision, my kids were bused to the local Catholic school with dozens of Italian and Portuguese children and were invited to lots of rec-room birthday parties. When I'd pick them up after the festivities, I was invariably invited to join the many celebrating aunts, uncles, and cousins for a glass of homemade wine and a slice or two of garlic-infused sausage. I had mixed feelings about these visits—much as I wanted to make friends with the parents of my children's pals, it was like having a conversation with a dozen Annas at once. It was easier with the men because they had usually learned enough English to communicate, but their wives stayed at home with their large families or, like Anna, helped other people with their cleaning and had less opportunity to learn or speak English.

Nevertheless, I never turned down an invitation, partly out of politeness and partly because I was curious. One evening, after

• NO GARLIC FOR FIDO •

Epicurean cats and dogs may love garlic as much as humans, but don't let them eat it. Even a bit of garlic in the leftover roast beef can cause hemolytic anemia in a small animal, destroying the red blood cells. The cells become rigid and rupture, then leak hemoglobin into the animal's urine.

I'd drunk two tumblers of homemade wine and liberally helped myself from a platter heaped with rounds of sausage, shavings of cheese, piles of glossy black olives and marinated artichoke hearts—new to me—and after I'd enthusiastically exclaimed over the little folds of salty pink ham I ate so ravenously, the father of the house asked if I'd like to see the *cantina*.

A SECOND kitchen in the basement! This was new to me, too, but I decided Anna must have had one as well—maybe all Italians did—for preserving and storing her tomatoes. There was a sink, a stove and big pots, a long counter, a utensil rack, and shelves and shelves of bottled tomatoes, pickles, fruits, and any number of vegetables. It was rather like the root cellar on my other grandma's farm. Hanging from the rafters were several dark pink hams, which the birthday boy's dad proudly told me he had prepared himself. "This is my prosciutto."

"Wow!" I said. "I had no idea you could *make* ham! I get mine sliced at the supermarket." Then I caught sight of a dozen or so hanging ropes of garlic.

"Did you grow all that?" I asked.

He laughed. "Yes." Did he think I was a pampered Canadian idiot who'd drunk too much of his wine? I was feeling a bit like one. He took down a rope and showed me how the bulbs, some pure white and some striped purple, like Anna's, were twisted together. "You just take the long stalks while they're still soft and tie them up," he said. Then he reached for a big knife and with his work-callused hands cut off a big bulb and handed it to me. "Will you take this for your *cucina?* You like the food so much, maybe you'd like to try it..."

He seemed anxious, as if he feared a gift of garlic was in bad taste, and I fell all over myself trying to tell him about Anna's garlic and how I'd been trying to find some like it in the stores, with no luck. I burbled on, thanking him profusely and feeling more than a little foolish.

But he must not have thought too badly of me because every few weeks for several months he sent an unblemished globe of garlic to school with his son, Aldo, for my son to pass along to me. I treasured the garlic and used it carefully, saving most of it for Anna's sauce.

DOWN TO EARTH
WITH GARLIC

How to Plant, Feed, Harvest, and Store Your Amazing Bulbs

---

*Planting garlic when the moon is below
the horizon and gathering it when it is in conjunction
prevents it from having an objectionable smell.*

PLINY THE ELDER

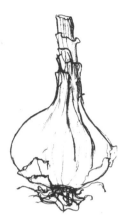

espite my vows and my desire for fresh, juicy garlic, I didn't try to grow my own. I was more involved with flowers than with vegetables, but deep down I was also intimidated by the idea of growing garlic. I knew nothing about it, and neither did my friends. I didn't want to ask Anna (the language problem), and I felt awkward about asking Aldo's dad. Then more white bulbs of garlic started appearing on grocery store shelves, and the urgency to grow it passed. My flower gardens expanded, and I had no space for garlic anyway.

But one day many years later, after Joe and I had parted and I had a new husband and a new house with flowers filling the front and back yards, my friend Judith came knocking on my door with a basket of huge, healthy cloves of garlic.

"You can plant what's in this basket or you can eat it," she said in her forthright way. "But since you have such a big garden now, I think it's time you grew it."

"But I don't know how to grow garlic. And where will I plant all these?" I moaned, pointing to the dozens of pristine white cloves. They were fat little crescents like the sections of a mandarin orange, fairly bursting with energy, and I could feel them calling to me. What I really wanted to do was eat them. But Judith had thrown down the gauntlet. It was time for me—garlic lover, gardener, cook—to grow the stuff.

"Okay, you can eat half of them," Judith conceded, taking a closer look at all the cottagey flowers jammed together in my garden. My philosophy is that planting close keeps the weeds out—or at least out of sight under the tightly spaced perennials— but Judith is a landscape designer and she knows an overplanted garden when she sees one. A little cloud passed over her face. "It's going to be hard to find space for even half a dozen cloves here," she said. "But we're going to make this work even if these aren't optimum conditions. Garlic is so tough they'll likely come up like gangbusters next year."

Judith is a positive person. I knew she was rethinking her decision to give me the garlic left over from her fall planting—a robust variety called 'Fish Lake #3,' which she'd ordered from Ted Maczka, an eccentric octogenarian grower in Ontario known as the Fish Lake Garlic Man (he'd sent the garlic to her in several waxed milk cartons)—but with her let's-deal-with-it attitude, she surveyed my garden and found its good points. "You've got lots of sun here, which is good—they like sun—and though your soil is pretty sandy, you've added lots of compost and it's looking okay.

Garlic isn't choosy, but it *does* prefer something a bit richer and loamier."

Her eagle eye found about a dozen spots with *praaw-ba-bly* enough space to allow the cloves to grow into bulbs. She waved her hand toward the spots, which weren't much wider than the coffee mug I was holding, between low-growing perennials like thyme and Carpathian bellflower (*Campanula carpatica*).

"These garlic guys have skinny leaves, and they need all the sun they can get," Judith said. "They need as little competition as possible, please." She raised her eyebrow. "Might you consider… aah, thinning out a couple of plants to make more room? Some of them are real spreaders."

I'd already thought of that and was ready to make a little space for my new visitors, especially if it meant lovely garlic to eat next year. Visions of Anna's and Aldo's dad's luscious garlic had started to dance in my head.

But on second thought, I couldn't dig up huge swaths of plants from my new front-yard garden to create optimum conditions for garlic, and in its present state my garden certainly didn't offer such conditions, as Judith had made clear. Still, she was right—it was time I grew some garlic. I'd been cooking with it for decades with little understanding of where it came from or how it was cultivated, even though I grew a few other vegetables, like tomatoes and beans and lettuces and herbs. I started them from seed in my basement and grew them in big pots on my driveway and my front steps, as well as in corners of my garden. I'd found places for them, hadn't I? I was also unhappy with the garlic generally sold in supermarkets—those small dried-up bulbs from China—and used garlic powder as a last resort.

Judith grew garlic successfully in her small city garden, so why couldn't I?

I BIT the bullet and pulled out a few filler annuals that weren't going to live much longer anyway, since it was late October. I also dug out some self-seeded lady's mantle and rampant gaura. I plunged a sharp trowel into the soil and excavated little holes for the garlic cloves. ("Pointed end up, please," Judith sang out. "Otherwise you'll have bent stems next year—I mean the garlic will..." She laughed.) It was worth getting rid of a few overgrown plants to try something new. Anyway, my garden needed a different look, which a few garlic plants might provide. And sometimes the best things you do are unplanned, even thrust upon you by others. Goodness knows I loved garlic's cousins, the ornamental alliums, which I grew in clumps and as single exclamation points among the flowers. And wow, if this experiment worked...

I have had a whole field of garlic planted...
so that when you come we may
be able to have many of your favorite dishes.
In a letter from BEATRICE D'ESTE, the Duchess of Milan,
to her sister Isabella, the Marchioness of Mantua, 1491

JUDITH AND I managed to squeeze in about two dozen cloves that day. (I ate the rest, but not that day and not all in one day. They were delicious.) After we finished planting we sat on the steps and celebrated with a glass of wine while Judith assured me that garlic was actually one of the easiest of plants to grow as long

• GARLIC'S WILD COUSINS •

Garlic grows wild, too, and some varieties are native to North America. *Allium canadense*, also called meadow garlic or wild shallot, grows mainly on the eastern part of the continent, from New Brunswick to Florida and west as far as Texas. Indigenous people relied on it as food and also used its juice as an insect repellent. It has narrow, grassy leaves and a dome of pink or white star-shaped flowers; its bulb is just over an inch (3 centimeters) in diameter and is covered with a dense network of brown fibers.

A. tricoccum, or "ramp," grows in many parts of the continent and is so prized for the mild garlic flavor of its bulb and wide, short leaves that it's an endangered species in the province of Quebec; in Maine, Rhode Island, and Tennessee, where annual festivals in its honor are common, it's considered a plant of "special concern." In the spring of 2011, more than 18,500 harvested plants on their way to various markets were seized by authorities in Quebec.

Allium vineale, sometimes called crow garlic, was introduced to North America from Europe and has invaded meadows and farm fields in many places, including Ontario, where it's listed as a weed. It has grasslike leaves and greenish-white, pink, or purplish flowers that grow in clusters. It's edible, though apparently not as tasty as other garlics. Cattle don't seem to mind its taste, however, and its flavor often affects dairy and beef products.

as you met most of its needs—which is true of all plants, when it comes down to it.

"In many ways garlic is like a tulip," she said. "You plant it in fall and it grows some roots and then lies underground for a cool sleep and wakes up when spring comes. The only difference is you don't dig up the tulips and eat them—well, there are more differences than that, but the principle is the same." She went on with more tips about growing, harvesting, and storing garlic. It sounded simple, and as we sipped and looked at the setting sun, I grew more and more confident that I'd have a lovely crop of garlic just like Judith's next summer. But Judith was thinking about what I needed to do to harvest at least *some* garlic.

"If you want to fertilize them, they like a little nitrogen," she said, going over a mental checklist. "I use blood meal mixed with the soil when I plant them." She advised me to dig them up when half the leaves had yellowed, and to make sure I stored them in a cool place.

"I guess I should keep what we don't eat right away in the fridge," I offered.

"Heavens no!" said Judith, looking horrified. "Put them in the fridge and they'll think it's winter again and start the growing process all over. They'll sprout! Keep them cool, not cold."

I figured I'd worry about that next year. "Now, what else?" Judith pondered. I topped up her glass. "Mmmm, yes—here's something important. In about mid-June you should cut off the scapes—the tall flower stems—so that the energy goes into bulb production. But damn, I love those scapes—they're the coolest things since TV. They're so entertaining as they weave around, curling and then straightening like magic. So I leave them on, and I don't find it affects my bulbs that much."

She turned to me with a wry grin. "Well, all this is according to me," she said and then drained her glass. "For the expert stuff, you might want to read up on raising garlic. Right now it's time for me to go."

"One more thing," she said as she backed out of the driveway. "Don't forget to lay on a mulch of some chopped leaves once the ground has frozen. You want to keep those little cloves warm and safe."

At that moment, even though my garlic cloves were safely tucked into their beds, I felt a twinge of nervous anticipation. I was a garlic virgin, left to nurture Judith's gifts on my own and unsure of how to go about it but filled with excitement about what was to come.

Oh, that miracle clove! Not only does garlic taste good,
it cures baldness and tennis elbow, too.
LAURIE BURROWS GRAD, food writer

OVER THE winter I completely forgot about those little cloves snuggled under the ground. I'm sure they didn't care. After all, they had a strong heritage of survival behind them, and they didn't need support from me.

My memory wasn't even jogged by the sight of garlic shoots peeking through the ground in spring. There were a couple of reasons for this. First, like too many gardeners who live to regret their laziness, I hadn't taken the time to mark the spots where Judith and I had planted the garlic the previous October. Second, I mistook the garlic shoots for the drumstick allium (A. *sphaerocephalon*) bulbs I'd planted weeks before we put in the garlic (which also weren't labeled, I might add). If I'd known what garlic looks like when it pokes its nose out of the ground, I would have recognized this as a bad sign. A. *sphaerocephalon* is a skinny ornamental with flowers like purple eggs at the end of long, wiry stems—dainty stems not at all like garlic's more robust ones. I like them planted singly or in threes as accent points throughout the garden, and I'd put in a couple of dozen. It was a few weeks before it dawned on me there were too many of them showing in my garden.

Could some of these be the garlic Judith and I planted? Is this what garlic looks like?

I phoned Judith right away. "This doesn't sound right," she said. "The shoots should be thicker, sort of stubby looking, but they could be small because they're so crowded. Never mind— give them some more room if you can, keep the ground weeded around them, give them a jolt of fertilizer, and you should harvest some small bulbs this summer."

Judith, ever the optimist. My confidence faded—this wasn't the gangbusters crop she had predicted. I didn't even know which plants were garlic and which were ornamental alliums. Then I came across a single fat garlic shoot I'd overlooked in an out-of-the-way space by a pathway. He was a beautiful boy—for how could I think of him as anything other than a boy, with his thick stem thrusting so strongly out of the ground? He grew vigorously, with a rounded fleshy top of grassy green over a vertically veined base, and within a few days he was taller. Once he reached thumb

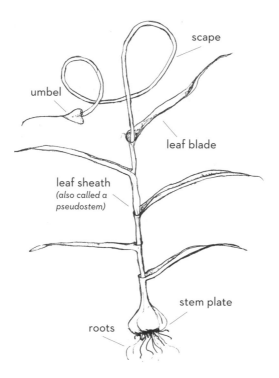

height, his fleshy top grew into a stem that lengthened and leafed out in even spaces, sending flat blades to float out laterally from perfectly incised cuts on the stem. Now this was garlic! Each leaf was placed exactly halfway around the stem from the one below it. My boy was a marvel of balanced design.

Like many beautiful boys, however, his appearance was deceiving. I'd done my homework and had read up on garlic, as Judith suggested, and I knew that this stem was not a stem at all but a tube or sheath of leaves that originated from the real stem underground, which doesn't look like any stem I've ever seen. It's a flat plate, called the stem plate, from which thin white roots grow downward as it pushes the leaf sheath upward. The garlic cloves—each of which contains all the elements needed to grow a whole new plant the next year, assuming we don't eat them—develop in a cluster around the leaf sheath on top of the stem plate, creating the bulb. When the bulb has been harvested and cured, the stem plate becomes the hard, scarred surface from which you snap off the cloves to use for dinner. I'd seen hundreds of garlic bulbs in my kitchen, and I never knew that hard base was actually the stem!

It was the leaves pushing up through the center of the sheath that accounted for my boy's quick growth—the second leaf emerged hastily from inside the first one, then the third from inside the second, like chorus girls popping out of a cake, rising higher and higher. As Judith had said, the leaves are important, even precious. Because there are so few—sometimes fewer than a dozen—losing just one leaf can reduce the size of the bulb by as much as 13 percent. A plant can lose leaves by amputation or by shade—hence the need to grow garlic with space around it and to weed assiduously.

My beautiful boy grew to a young man, and I checked him carefully every few days, weeding around him and cutting away potentially interfering perennials. I watched his siblings, too—no favoritism here, even though I was banking on my young man to make me a successful garlic grower, even if it was only of one plant. I did as much as I could for the others when I could find them in my crowded garden, digging out the plants around them, making sure they had enough water. Unfortunately, my garden had not been the right place for them from the beginning, and it was a losing battle. They remained skinny Minnies, though they all grew scapes because they were from the hardneck family of garlics. As already mentioned, garlic comes in two types—hardneck (*Allium sativum* var. *ophioscorodon*), which is closer to the ancient type and grows a scape that curls as it matures, and softneck (*Allium sativum* var. *sativum*). Hardneck types produce a single row of six to eleven cloves, which cluster around its underground base. Softneck garlic, on the other hand, grows with no theatrics—and by that I mean no graceful, curling flower scapes. It is a shorter plant, and its bulb produces several rows of cloves, larger ones in an outer row and smaller ones inside them, closer to the leaf sheath, sometimes as many as twenty-four. Softneck garlic is the choice of large-scale commercial growers because it grows well in California and other warmer climates, which produce large quantities for sale and export; growers don't need to remove the scapes, which would add to production costs; and softneck garlic usually can be stored longer than hardneck varieties. Softneck garlic is the one used for braiding because the stalk is pliable enough to manipulate.

Garlic completely conquers lassitude, catarrh,
rheumatism of the arms and back, and epilepsy.
THE BOWER MANUSCRIPT

BUT MAN, Judith was right. Those scapes on the hardnecks were indeed entertaining. I'd heard of the fields of sunflowers in France whose yellow faces follow the sun from morning to night, but this natural phenomenon of plant movement was happening, albeit in a different time frame, in my own front yard! Small and skinny as they were, the scapes still put on a great show, coiling gracefully downward over a week's time, their umbels like flamingo beaks searching the sea for food, then straightening out and pointing toward the heavens. They added an offbeat presence to my garden of busty flowers, and people taking post-prandial walks down our street often stopped to ask what they were. I decided to let most of the scapes grow to maturity, as Judith did, but I decapitated some when they started to straighten out, including my boy's. This was a few years before scapes became a gourmand's delight, so I was ignorant of their culinary value and tossed them onto the compost heap. I hoped trimming them off would allow a few struggling plants to develop nice big bulbs for me to eat.

Well, it didn't. Harvest time came, and I carefully dug up the bulbs and found that most of them were "rounds," garlicspeak for bulbs composed of a single clove, but bigger than the ones in a multicloved bulb. There's nothing wrong with rounds. They taste good—you just don't get as much garlic. Some of my bulbs had two small cloves, nowhere near the usual yield for 'Fish Lake #3,' which normally produces four to six. Nevertheless, I washed the rounds off carefully, dried them in the sun, and hung all ten of them from a rafter in the garage. Once they were cured they kept me in garlic for about two weeks.

Ah, but would my young man fulfill my dream? I held my breath as I approached him near the end of July; he looked older and a little droopy, with mostly dried, tan-colored leaves. I carefully put my trowel in the ground and dug him up. He was gorgeous! Not huge, but handsome—maybe the diameter of an

Oreo with three fat cloves around his nearly dried leaf sheath. Best of all, he was proof I might eventually grow a successful crop of good garlic.

I trimmed his roots and hung him in a special spot in the garage as he dried and cured. Then I cut his stem off just above his neck and put him on a shelf in the kitchen where I could admire him as I cooked. His dry, taut skin looked pearly white, and his body was beautifully rounded. I admired him for many weeks, and then I could wait no longer.

I ate him.

I can't get enough garlic!

TED WILLIAMS

I HAVE a confession to make: I didn't plant garlic at all for the next few years.

But about four years after my disappointing first try, I watched with interest as dozens of skinny garlic plants sprang up all over our front garden. Were these the offspring of Judith's garlic? Why had they waited so long? As far as I knew, modern garlic had lost the ability to set seed. Was a miracle occurring here, in my own garden?

No, there was a simpler explanation. It wasn't seed; it was the bulbils, those curious tiny clove look-alikes growing among the little flowers in the umbels, doing what they'd been programmed to do. They'd blown far and wide in my garden, and although it had taken them a few growing seasons, they were producing new plants. In late July I dug most of them up to see how they were doing and discovered a crop of small but deliciously juicy rounds. I left the rest to grow the following year, when I actually harvested some bulbs—small ones, to be sure, but some had three cloves. The next year they were bigger still.

It was enough to give me garlic fever.

Our front garden was clearly not the place to grow great garlic, so I decided to transform our last scrap of grass in the back into a thyme patch, leaving enough growing room between the new thyme plants for twenty-four garlic plants. The garlic I ordered from the website of a West Coast grower was big and luscious, and I bought more at a local September garlic fair—'Persian Star,' 'Rosewood,' 'Dan's Russian,' 'Mount Currie,' 'Fish Lake #3,' and others—to plant as well as to store and eat over the winter. I've planted two garlic crops in that space now, and they were as easy to grow and as problem free as anything I've ever grown. I will admit the bulbs aren't as big as I'd like, but they're juicy and hot and a hundred times better than the small, dried-up Chinese store-bought variety. I figure I'm still learning how to put into practice all the little tips I've picked up, and soon I'll be growing garlic like what I see at the fairs, the kind that make a statement in your garlic jar.

HOW TO GROW GARLIC

Everyone from Judith to the speakers at garlic fairs and the authors of the books I'd read had assured me that growing garlic was rewardingly easy. The simple fact is that garlic is a happy, adaptable plant that grows in many places in the world and does well in temperate areas of North America, which is most of it. It has a strong life force and wants to survive. It will sometimes change its habits to suit the conditions it faces, as when centuries ago the hardnecks evolved into softnecks in the Mediterranean area and created a new kind of garlic. I love this unsung little plant!

Garlic takes nine months to reach fruition, and in almost every part of North America it's best planted in fall, three or four weeks before hard frost, so that it has time to develop some root growth before winter comes. Then it needs a period of cold to fully develop its bulb. Hardnecks, such as the popular Rocamboles, for example, prefer frosty winters and yield poorly without a period of vernalization, but there are always exceptions. A man southwest of Abilene, Texas, reported successfully growing a couple of Purple Stripe hardnecks in his garden, one named 'Siberian' just to make sure we know it likes the cold. The normally scapeless softneck cultivars do best in mild winters, but some of them, such as those of the Silverskin subgroup, do fine in colder areas where—just to demonstrate their adaptable natures— they occasionally grow a scape. (For help with what varieties to plant in your part of the world, see "A Garlic Primer.")

Nevertheless, garlic needs some cool weather to develop the bulb, and some types like it colder than others. For example, the softneck garlic grown in California has adapted to milder winters but still needs chilly January or February weather to grow full cloves; the types grown in Central Asia, however, require really harsh winters to produce them. In places like North Africa and South Asia, where winter doesn't exist at all, multicloved bulbs simply don't form. In those parts, garlic is grown for its leaves, which are tasty too.

• BABIES LIKE GARLIC, TOO •

Many breast-feeding mothers avoid eating garlic because they fear it will upset their babies, but a couple of studies by Julie Mennella and Gary Beauchamp of the Monell Chemical Senses Center in Philadelphia, and quoted by Eric Block in his book *Garlic and Other Alliums*, suggest that infants may be attracted to garlic. The studies, done in 1991 and 1993, indicated that babies "remained attached to the breast for longer periods of time, sucked more when the milk smelled like garlic, and ingested more milk as well." The babies in the study who had not been exposed to garlic in their mothers' milk spent more time breast-feeding after their mothers consumed garlic capsules.

AS I discovered in my garden, if garlic is left in the ground year after year, the bulbs become ever smaller but more numerous. This is because each clove grows a new plant, and the plants become so crowded that the bulbs can't reach a good size. Plants that grow from scattered bulbils take about three years to grow large enough to produce single, smallish rounds, but sometimes leaving the scapes on and allowing garlic to reproduce through bulbils is a way to enjoy the presence of graceful scapes in the garden as well as a taste of fresh, homegrown garlic.

SELECTING THE SITE

Garlic likes full sun. It's not too difficult to meet this requirement, since the period from early spring into mid to late July, the general harvest time in most parts of the continent, is usually the sunniest time of the year, with the longest days. But plant in an open area with maximum sunshine and keep the area free of even small weeds, since even they can shade the slender garlic leaves.

Garlic is usually planted in rows in the vegetable garden, but because it's such a dramatic plant with ornamental attractions I see no reason why you can't plant it in open areas of a sunny perennial border, singly for architectural interest or in groups of one variety each. (Need I remind you to label the spots where you bury the cloves?) In our back bed I plant garlic in circular groups of one variety, with each circle about 18 inches (half a meter) away from low perennials. They've grown happily that way for two seasons, though I know that's not going to last. I'll have to dig up another part of our garden or rent an allotment garden if I want to continue to feed my garlic obsession.

One other consideration in choosing a site: like tomatoes and other plants in the Solanaceae family, garlic crops shouldn't be planted in the same place every year. This suggestion isn't especially practical in a small home garden, but if you can plant garlic on the other side of the vegetable plot the following year, you should be able to avoid a buildup of pathogens or pests in the soil.

PREPARING THE SOIL

Garlic may have originated in thin, rocky soils centuries ago, but no one was demanding a lot of it back then. It was surviving, not thriving, hanging on and establishing itself as the tough little plant it's turned out to be. These days we want it to produce fat bulbs, so we must provide it with friable soil that drains well but is rich in organic matter. A neutral to slightly acidic pH level (6 to 7.5) is perfect. If you want to test your soil, kits are usually available at garden centers or through the local agricultural office. Most soils sit between pH 5 and 9, however, so yours is not likely a problem.

If I were preparing a garlic bed a year in advance—the best way to do it—in the fall I'd dig in some grass clippings, chopped leaves, and vegetable trimmings from the kitchen, without putting them through the composting process. Mixed well with the existing soil, they'll break down for the following fall's planting. But if you're a last-minute person, like me, and you decide you want to plant garlic *now*, incorporate a good layer of compost or well-rotted manure and mix it in to a depth of about 6 inches (15 centimeters).

PLANTING

Some of the garlic cloves I planted with Judith had only 3 inches (7.5 centimeters) of soil around them—no wonder they grew up to be midgets! Most garlic should be planted 4 to 6 inches (10 to 15 centimeters) apart; larger varieties, such as the Porcelain group, need 6 inches (15 centimeters), so you should know your variety. If you're planting in rows, space them no less than 8 inches (20 centimeters) apart so that the rows don't shade each other. Rows can be wider, of course, and spacing will depend on convenience, such as location of access pathways.

Don't buy separate cloves to plant—it's better to start with whole bulbs and separate the cloves just before planting. Separated cloves may have small cuts or loosened skins, which could make them vulnerable to viruses or bacteria. Twist the bulbs gently or pry off the cloves, being careful not to nick them

• SPRING PLANTING OPTION •

Even in Gilroy, California, the garlic capital of the world, garlic is planted in fall so that the seed cloves experience enough cool weather to produce good-sized bulbs. But gardeners like to experiment, and many try spring planting to see what happens. If you want to try, choose softneck cultivars in the Artichoke or Silverskin subgroups and prechill cloves for three weeks at 45 to 50°F (7 to 10°C) to break dormancy. Plant in February or early March.

In the southern United States or other warm-winter areas, spring planting of prechilled bulbs is sometimes the only option. It also can work where winters are so frigid that cloves tend to freeze in the ground: prepare holes before freeze-up and plant cloves during an early spring thaw, covering with purchased potting soil. Spring-planted garlic generally produces smaller bulbs.

or tear off their papery skin. Plant the cloves, pointed end up, in holes about 3 inches (7.5 centimeters) deep. There should be about 2 inches (5 centimeters) of soil between the tops and the soil surface. "If you plant them upside down they'll end up in China!" said Ted Maczka, the Fish Lake Garlic Man, at a garlic fair seminar, laughing at his joke until the garlic bulbs glued to his visored cap shook dangerously. "Then the Chinese will sell them all back to us."

Ted may have retired to a seniors' home, but he frequently returns to his garlic farm in Ontario's Prince Edward County to play classical music to his plants. "They show up early through the snow in spring looking for the beautiful music," he says. He talks to them, too, because they're living things with an energy flow and they like being included in the conversation.

IF YOU live a distance north or south of the forty-ninth parallel or the Great Lakes, the rules change. Plant a little deeper the farther north you live, a little shallower if you're in a more southern climate. In severely cold climates, cover the cloves with as much as 4 inches (10 centimeters) of soil (plus a winter blanket of mulch); in California an inch (2 centimeters) should suffice. But don't lose too much sleep over planting depths—if you plant too deep the shoots may take longer to pop through the earth in spring, but they'll catch up once the weather is warm.

Many garlic growers say the most successful seed cloves don't come from the biggest bulbs; in fact large seed cloves don't ensure a crop of big bulbs the following year. But really small cloves aren't ideal either; they may not grow bulbs that are properly segmented. Use only the larger outer cloves of softneck varieties for seed. "Eat the biggest and the smallest," says Ted Maczka. "Plant the middle-sized ones."

WATERING

Garlic that doesn't get enough to drink suffers stress and may start to produce bulbs early, resulting in smaller cloves and bulbs. The bulbs may shatter at harvest, too, meaning the skins split and leave the cloves underneath vulnerable to bacteria and rotting. Split skin is okay if you have a small crop and expect to eat it within a few weeks, but the bulbs won't store successfully; nor, as mentioned, should you use them as seed stock.

Watering requires a commonsense approach. Plants need enough for healthy growth, but they shouldn't be sitting in puddles. An inch or two (2.5 to 5 centimeters) of water a week is ideal, applied with a soaker hose or sprinkler in the morning if there hasn't been enough rain. Give the plants a deep watering rather than a surface sprinkling. Garlic may be shallow rooted, but the soil must be damp enough deeply enough to prevent it from drying out quickly. Sandy soil needs to be watched because it dries out fast in hot, sunny weather.

Make sure the soil is damp when you plant the cloves so that the roots can begin to grow immediately—languishing in dry soil makes them prone to disease or deterioration. When harvest time approaches, garlic needs less water so that growth will slow and the bulbs can mature. I never pray for rain after the middle of July, and in a heavy downpour I'm tempted to rush into the garden and hold an umbrella over the garlic patch to protect the plants from soggy soil that might encourage rot. There's not much you can do about an unwelcome rainfall, but you can withhold extra irrigation via the sprinkler.

USING FERTILIZER

Loamy soil high in organic matter, which holds moisture but doesn't get waterlogged, is more important than a truckload of fertilizer. If any fertilizer is needed, it will be nitrogen, as my oracle Judith advised. Plants lacking nitrogen look poorly—during the growing season, they show weakened vigor and a general yellowing, and they produce small bulbs earlier than normal. Judith follows the general rule and mixes blood meal with the soil when she's planting the cloves, then applies it as a side dressing a couple of times during the season.

Nitrogen encourages foliage growth and can slow bulb formation near harvest time, so hold off on fertilizer altogether as harvest approaches.

Because it's a root crop, garlic may also benefit from a little potassium. Wood ashes are a good organic form.

DEALING WITH PESTS AND DISEASES

There's something to be said for being smelly and strong tasting— it chases away diseases and pests. For millennia garlic's sulfurous compounds have defended it against plant-eating pests and have poisoned strains of fungi and bacteria that dared invade its skin. But garlic isn't immune to everything, and the list of its biological enemies below may suggest that garlic isn't all that tough. Still, most of its threats aren't deadly and can be controlled by good garden practices, such as removing and destroying plants that look sick, avoiding too much watering and subsequent soggy soil and humid air, and planting only healthy, unblemished cloves with intact skins. Crop rotation (changing the planting location) also helps prevent the spread of viruses and fungi, and it's always a good idea when you trim or deadhead neighboring plants to remove plant debris from the area in case it's harboring bugs or disease.

VIRUSES ARE common, and although most aren't fatal, they will affect a plant's vigor. Symptoms of viruses can include striping,

• GARLIC, THE BUG KILLER OF THE FUTURE? •

Now that we're aware of the dangers of using poisonous chemicals to kill garden pests, garlic may come into its own as a nature-friendly pesticide. For centuries garlic, onions, and leeks have protected themselves by releasing sulfur compounds into the air or the soil—or into the mouths of insects that bite them. Our ancestors knew this and used garlic as an insecticide and companion plant, and contemporary tests of oils and extracts of alliums against nematodes, beetles, mites, ticks, and more have produced impressive results. Garlic oil has also been shown to be toxic to larvae of the mosquito, which spreads malaria, dengue fever, West Nile virus, yellow fever, encephalitis, and other diseases.

streaking, or mottling on the leaves and twisted or stunted leaves, and if one plant has a virus, it's likely to soon spread to others via aphids or thrips. Practice prevention: keep plants healthy and unstressed by making sure they have enough water and a fertile soil.

A couple of stem rots caused by soilborne fungi in the *Fusarium* genus can affect the stem plate, leaving it with rotted roots, brownish discoloration, or lesions with a reddish fringe. Early symptoms include yellowing leaf tips and shoot dieback, though sometimes leaves show no symptoms at all. Blue mold, caused by various strains of *Penicillium* molds, can enter bulbs through damage during storage or can invade damaged cloves separated from the mother bulb too long before planting. Infected

---

• HOMEMADE BUG DETERRENT •

To deter whiteflies, aphids, beetles, and mosquitoes, try this garlic spray. Be sure to completely cover the plant, including the undersides of the leaves.

4 ounces	garlic extract
a few drops	dish soap or insecticidal soap
1 quart	water

Blend together and strain through cheesecloth. Dilute ten times and spray on plants, including undersides of leaves. No garlic extract? Blend a whole bulb of garlic with 2 cups of water, allow to sit for a day, and strain. Add a few drops of dish soap and dilute with 1 gallon of water.

---

cloves may not grow or may produce weak plants with yellow leaves, though strong plants often overcome the disease. An infected bulb can easily spread the mold to its neighbors in storage.

Pink root, which is caused by a fungus active in temperatures above 75°F (24°C), attacks the plant's roots, turning them pink. You might see a little leaf browning, but the plant doesn't usually die. Pink root may reduce crop yields, however.

Rust, another fungus, shows up as yellow or white spots or streaks on leaves followed by orange pustules filled with orange spores. If the disease worsens, black pustules appear. High humidity and low rainfall encourage the disease, but, oddly, warm weather (above 75°F, or 24°C) or temperature below 50°F (10°C) inhibits it. Although rust is not often a problem, it will spread easily by wind if it gets a foothold—a late-1990s outbreak in California severely reduced crop yields. Again, prevention is key. Keep plants healthy and unstressed, without either too much or too little water, and avoid applying too much nitrogen.

WHITE ROT, caused by *Sclerotium cepivorum*, has been responsible for many crop losses in the United States and other parts of the world. It also affects other members of the *Allium* genus. It starts as a fluffy white mycelium—a network of branching, threadlike spores—on the stem plate, which then advances up the plant. Growth is stunted, and leaves yellow and die. If only one plant appears to be infected, both it and the surrounding soil should be dug up and removed and the adjacent soil fumigated. But once the fungus has become established, alliums cannot be grown on the site for many years.

When a cow has been three nights with almost no grass,
give her a preparation of two parts grass to one part garlic stalks.
A Brahmin can then partake of her milk and maintain propriety.
THE BOWER MANUSCRIPT

INSECTS THAT affect garlic include mites, and an infestation can destroy a bulb. Onion maggots and thrips sometimes attack garlic; the maggots bore into the bulbs, and the thrips chew on the precious leaves. Microscopic nematodes, or eelworms, eat garlic, onions, leeks, and chives, as well as celery and parsley. The nematodes are so tiny they're invisible. In severe cases the bulb may separate from the underground stem and turn into a pulpy mass—sometimes when you try to harvest the bulb it's not there.

Planting only healthy, unblemished bulbs is the best way to prevent nematodes, but pouring hot water over cloves you're about to plant might kill the little devils.

There's one bug that's scaring the garden gloves off garlic growers in eastern Canada these days: the leek moth, *Acrolepiopsis assectella*. It's an uninvited European species that probably made its way to Canada on infected plant material, and it has been significantly damaging garlic crops in eastern Ontario, southern Quebec, and Prince Edward Island since it appeared in the Ottawa area in 1993, tunneling into and eating the leaves, scapes, and bulbs. It's now reported in upper New York State. In March 2010 the Canadian Food Inspection Agency released a parasitic wasp in hopes it would control the moth, but results won't be known for several years.

If you live in these areas and discover the leek moth, Paul Pospisil of the *Garlic News* suggests an old-fashioned approach to control: checking for cocoons and larvae daily and crushing them by hand to reduce the population. The larvae can reach just over half an inch (1.4 centimeters) in length and are yellowish-green with pale brown heads and eight gray spots on each abdominal segment. Adult moths are reddish-brown, about one-quarter inch (0.6 centimeters) long, with a white triangular mark in the middle of the folded wings; hind wings are heavily fringed and pale gray to black.

Gophers love garlic and will eat the whole crop if they can. Chester Aaron, who grows garlic in Sonoma County, California, and is the author of *The Great Garlic Book, Garlic Is Life, Garlic Kisses*, and more, protects his garlic by growing it in raised beds framed with wood and set on chicken wire. Grasshoppers can be a threat: in Texas it was reported that a heavy infestation in 2004 destroyed 24,000 plants; the varmints ate the tops and then somehow dug into the ground to get at the succulent bulbs. It's impossible to protect against an army of grasshoppers, but for a smaller invasion Ted Meredith, author of *The Complete Book of Garlic*, suggests that floating row covers (plastic or fabric stretched over the bed on metal hoops, available at garden supply stores) could mount a defense for a short period. Row covers retain heat and if left on too long could bring the plants to maturity too soon.

How to Harvest and Store Your Bulbs

HARVESTING

A few weeks before you dig up mature hardneck bulbs, remove the scapes so that the plant can put all of its energy into bulb development—some growers say that leaving them on can reduce the yield of a field of garlic by as much as 33 percent. Snip them off with scissors or carefully snap them off where you see a white or pinkish spot on the stem.

Digging up the bulbs is the most fun of all, but knowing exactly when to do it can seem complicated. With all garlic, both hardneck and softneck, if you harvest too early the bulbs won't have reached optimum growth and flavor; too late and they will have burst their wrappers and left themselves vulnerable to bacteria, which would spell doom for successful storing. The bulbs might even have separated, leaving them useless for planting, although you could eat them right away.

Garlic should be harvested when some of the leaves are still green and some have browned, but exactly how many of each is a matter of discussion among some garlic growers. Some say half of the leaves should be brown; others say much more than half is desirable. Still others say the best time is when half of the leaves are half browned. Got it? It does get complicated, perhaps unnecessarily so. Commercial growers in California leave their softneck garlic in the ground till the tops brown and collapse, because they're easier to harvest with no green stems. I start with the half-and-half-of-total-leaves formula and then follow my instincts. If the plant is still looking too perky, even though half the leaves seem nicely browned, I leave it in a few more days.

Generally speaking, most softneck garlic and the Asiatics, Turbans, and Creoles—which sometimes grow a short scape (it depends on their environment or their ancestry)—are content to stay in the ground longer than other hardnecks. There are no hard-and-fast rules for garlic, but it is this flexibility that makes it an easy plant to raise, despite all these caveats.

Dig plants individually, using a trowel or a fork to loosen the soil before you gently pull them up. Brush loose dirt off newly dug cloves or let it dry and fall off, but wash off sticky clay right away, being sure to dry off the cloves and hang them upside down so that water doesn't enter the neck of the bulb. I trim off the roots at this point, but some gardeners leave them on until the final cleaning.

Let the bulbs lie uncrowded in a cool, shaded area, on a wire rack or a slotted surface, for a week or so. (I leave mine on the slatted bench built into our deck under an overhead trellis, and amazingly the raccoons leave them alone. I guess, unlike gophers, they haven't discovered the gourmet delights of garlic.) Then brush off the rest of the dried soil—an artist's paintbrush or a toothbrush works well—and tie the stems in small labeled bunches of one variety. Hang them in your garage or garden shed or on a rack in a protected place. They should cure for a few weeks to develop their flavor—four is a rough guideline, but two weeks is okay. It depends on how humid your climate is. Once the leaves and stems are quite brown and dead, the time is ripe to prepare your garlic for long-term storage.

If I play with garlic, my hands are bound to stink.

POMPONIUS, 110–132 BC

STORING

This is the knottiest problem for home growers who don't have a cold cellar and want to store garlic for several months. Ideally, garlic you want to keep into the winter should be stored at 56 to 59°F (13 to 15°C) with low humidity—45 to 50 percent. A wine cellar is perfect. So, strangely enough, is my bedroom closet, which is next to an outer wall in our older house; there are some advantages to poor insulation. I discovered this quite by accident when I wondered why my clothes were so cold and stuck a thermometer on the floor of the closet. My garlic lasts for six to eight months there, depending on variety.

But garlic will last for three or four months under a wider range of temperatures, including cool room temperature, about 68°F (20°C). As with other root vegetables, warm temperatures dry out the cloves and humidity causes mold to develop. Some commercial growers say bulbs can be stored at the freezing point and a slightly higher humidity with good results. One experiment kept bulbs beautifully at exactly 27°F (−3°C) for eight months, and they stayed in good condition for up to two months after coming to room temperature. But I can't control my freezer that precisely, so mine won't be coming out of the closet. Whatever you do, don't store garlic in the fridge. Refrigerators hit that magic range from 40 to 50°F (5 to 10°C) where garlic decides it's early spring and time to sprout. Sprouted garlic is edible but past its prime, especially if the sprout has grown to an inch (2.5 centimeters) or more.

Garlic needs air circulation, too, so don't store it in paper bags. Most mail-order growers send the bulbs in mesh bags, which are ideal; I also save onion bags from the grocery store, and in a pinch I've used the legs of panty hose, with the feet cut out and tied off.

Storing garlic for planting in the fall is easy; it can be kept at anywhere from 50°F (10°C) to room temperature until it's time to pop the cloves into the ground.

Garlic is at its juiciest when first harvested, and the flavor gets richer during storage. But there is a cutoff point when it starts to lose its bloom—just like carrots or potatoes stored too long. Generally speaking, hardnecks don't last as long as softnecks, and their flavor peaks earlier. The Rocamboles and Purple Stripes should be eaten sooner than, say, the Silverskins. But this is general: the Creoles, one of the three mentioned earlier that are officially grouped as hardnecks yet grow only a short scape, if any, are among the longest lasting of garlic varieties—they'll keep for up to a year in the right conditions. Labels are advisable when storing garlic. Again, for help with what to plant, plus tasting notes for a few varieties, see "A Garlic Primer."

CELEBRATING GARLIC

Two Festivals and a Universal Passion for Garlic

——————— • ———————

*The air of Provence is impregnated
with the aroma of garlic,
which makes it very healthful to breathe.*

ALEXANDRE DUMAS

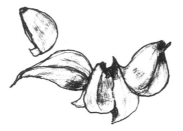

*F*or *a couple* of years I haunted nearby garlic fairs, sitting on hard benches in tents to hear lectures on the history, folklore, and medicinal value of garlic, jotting down growing and harvesting advice, watching cooking and braiding demonstrations, lunching on garlic sausage and garlic burgers, and sampling exotica like garlic fudge. I brought home jars of pickled garlic and garlic chutney and luscious garlic cultivars to eat and plant.

But I wanted more. The local fairs I was going to were all starting to look the same. I wanted to go to some really big ones, like the monster three-day bash held in Gilroy, California, at the end of July. I wanted to see what other countries' festivals had to offer. And I wanted to find a certain pink garlic I'd been reading about, Ail Rose de Lautrec, reputedly a gently pleasing variety with amazing storage qualities and satiny pink skin.

To add to the allure of its taste, Lautrec pink garlic has a romantic past. It first appeared in the French village in the mid-Pyrenees in the Middle Ages, when a mysterious traveler who didn't have enough francs to pay for his lodging offered the innkeeper a few bulbs of a lovely rose-pink garlic instead. The innkeeper planted it, and news of the garlic's superior taste and keeping qualities spread, though for hundreds of years it was grown only in small quantities in the kitchen gardens of the village. Today it's grown around the village under the strictest of regulations, using selected growers who have to follow the rules or else, and the village holds a garlic fair the first Friday of every August to celebrate it. But no one at any of the garlic fairs I attended had ever heard of it. I'd have to go to France to find it, and as a garlic-growing convert I was prepared to make the sacrifice.

So during a lull in the conversation at a family dinner one night, I announced to the group at large that I'd be going to the Gilroy Garlic Festival in California at the end of July and the Fête de l'Ail Rose in France in early August, and that the no-expenses-paid position of traveling companion for both these occasions was up for grabs.

There was a short pause and then my daughter, Suzy, put up her hand.

"I'll take Gilroy," she said. "It sounds like a blast."

I kept the bidding open, but no one else volunteered that evening. After only a minimum of arm-twisting, Chris later agreed to accompany me to France. Two trips to destinations thousands of miles apart in the space of ten days—it was an ambitious project, I realized. But it didn't take me long to realize I was doing more than gathering facts about garlic. I was learning how universal is the passion for this ancient vegetable and how differently people celebrate it.

There is no such thing as a little garlic.

ARTHUR BAER

"DO I smell garlic? Or am I imagining things just because we're in Gilroy?" asks Suzy, rolling down the car window and sniffing the air. We've just come off Highway 101 and are cruising into town, heading for our bed-and-breakfast before taking in the first day of the Gilroy Garlic Festival, the biggest one in the world.

"You're not imagining it—I smell it too," I say, drawing a deep, delicious breath. The mouthwatering aroma is all around us, as if some chef in the sky is cooking up a giant casserole of chicken with forty thousand cloves of garlic. But where is it coming from?

Gilroy's streets are lined with pretty, low-slung houses with lush-looking gardens, but as far as I can see there isn't a garlic plant in any of them. There's plenty in the fields outside town, regiments of them growing in endless rows, but garlic plants with their feet still in the earth don't give off a brain-blowing aroma like this. It seems a fitting introduction to a weekend of garlic overload.

Gilroy is an old town, incorporated in 1870, and now a pleasant, middle-class city half an hour inland from the Pacific Ocean and about a ninety-minute drive south of San Francisco. It has a well-dressed, conservative American look that seems at odds with the pervasive perfume of garlic, and right now it's almost deserted.

"Maybe everyone's at the festival," Suzy says. We follow a few people with folding chairs and sun hats to Christmas Hill Park, where the three-day festival has just got started. Gilroy boldly advertises itself as the garlic capital of the world, though this isn't technically true; Gilroy Foods (the source of that tantalizing smell, it turns out) may be the biggest processor of garlic in the world—pickled, minced, roasted, granulated, powdered, and more—but the United States ranks only sixth in the production of fresh garlic, behind China, India, South Korea, Egypt, and Russia. Still, garlic is the city's lifeblood, and the festival has put Gilroy (population 52,027 at last count) on the map. It's been run with good old American know-how since 1979, with mainly volunteer help—a thousand people the first year and about four thousand each year since—and almost everyone in town has volunteered at some point. The first year the organizing committee hoped to attract five thousand people, and three times that many showed up. They ran out of food and had to send out for shrimp and calamari, butter and bread to feed the hordes. (They had plenty of garlic.)

NO ONE expected such success—least of all the mayor at the time. Before the first festival the organizing committee enthusiastically approached him to ask for city sponsorship, and he said no, a garlic festival was a bizarre idea and the city wouldn't *think* of supporting it. So the committee went ahead on its own. The mayor refused to attend the festival. Every year since then about a hundred thousand people—twice the population of Gilroy—have shown up the last weekend in July to eat, drink, dance, and celebrate garlic.

• TURNING HOURS INTO DOLLARS •

The nonprofit Gilroy Garlic Festival does more than promote garlic: it raises money for local charities through general admission, Gourmet Alley foods, and booth rentals. More than $8 million has been raised since 1979. In addition, each person volunteering at the festival "earns" a theoretical wage based on hours worked, which is then donated to the charity of the volunteer's choice. In recent years this has ranged from $85.35 given to a wildlife education center to more than $10,000 to Gilroy High School's choir.

By the time Suzy and I get to the parking lot, a carnival atmosphere has appeared from nowhere. We hear the noise: a brass band here, a thrumming bass over there, people shouting, laughter. We see the peaks of tents and towering red flames shooting into the air. Within minutes we're caught up in the throng—seniors, moms and dads with kids in strollers, couples holding hands, teenagers running and pushing their way to one of the bands playing on three open-air stages. The crowds sweep us along to Gourmet Alley, the food stalls and cooking area that are the heart of the festival.

And they say Friday, today, is the festival's least busy day.

This time we see as well as smell lots of garlic, bowls of it chopped and waiting to be stirred into the huge pans and cauldrons sitting over open flames on long gas barbecue racks. The crowd pushes up against the metal barrier to watch the Pyro

Chefs, two festival regulars, put on their show. With theatrical flourish they shake giant pans filled with hundreds of shrimp and calamari. Flames lick the sides of the pans, moving higher and higher. There's a hush—the crowd knows what's coming—the chefs tip the pans ever so slightly, and *whoosh!* Bright orange flames leap into the air and billow dangerously near the tented roof. "*Woooo,*" gasps the crowd, pulling back from the barrier. This is showbiz.

"Wow," says Suzy. "Now I know why those guys are wearing dark glasses—they'd have no eyelashes without them."

What garlic is to food, insanity is to art.

AUGUSTUS SAINT-GAUDENS

THE BARBECUES were lit a couple of hours earlier in a ceremony befitting the Olympics. From a giant flaming garlic bulb in the center of the park, a bamboo garden torch was lit by the festival president and passed to various important dignitaries, then to Miss Gilroy Garlic Festival, who carried it to Mr. Garlic, a beautifully whiskered gentleman wearing the kind of getup even the most loving grandfather wouldn't be caught dead in on Halloween: a pouffy white garlic-shaped dress that bared his hairy white shoulders and legs, and a wide-brimmed garlic-laden straw hat. Mr. Garlic held the torch aloft for all to see as he proudly carried it to Gourmet Alley and ceremoniously lit the barbecues, to much applause.

The smell of garlic and onions, browning steak, and roasting peppers is making Suzy and me crazy, so we join the lineup for a combination plate, which seems like a good way to sample the variety Gourmet Alley offers. Our plastic plates are piled high, and not with mere samples. Mine holds a fat garlic sausage with grilled sweet peppers on a bun, a big ladle of small shrimp swimming in sauce, some chicken stir-fry, a big hunk of oozing garlic bread. Suzy's has a generous helping of calamari, a pile of pasta con pesto, half a pepper-steak sandwich, and the garlic bread. We eat perched uncomfortably on a bale of hay vacated by a couple of women who've just cleaned their plates; they wave us over when they see us holding our plates aloft and peering around hopefully.

As Grandma used to say, our eyes are bigger than our stomachs. It's too much food and too much garlic, even for garlic lovers, and except for the delicious, juicy sausage, the food is a tad overcooked—a problem with mass production, I know. But like those garlic-eating ancient Roman soldiers, we're well fortified for the afternoon's foray. We walk out onto the grounds, ready for whatever awaits us.

The grounds are anthills of activity, tents and booths as far as my squinting eyes can see. People from almost every community between San Francisco and San Diego are here, plus more from Denver and Detroit, Orlando and Austin, and Liverpool, England, and Toronto, Canada, buying T-shirts, posters, garlic graters, leather handbags, cookbooks, historic framed photos of old America, jewelry and wineglasses etched with "Gilroy Garlic Festival 2010." The food vendors set up around the periphery sell more garlic-laden dishes: beef teriyaki, blackened shrimp with rice, BBQ ribs, Cajun crawdads, and garlic-fried green tomatoes. We needn't worry where to find a bite to eat over the next couple of days.

Suzy heads for the big Garlic Mercantile tent for a look at its wares, and I move through the crowds and in and out of booths selling sterling silver toe rings, nifty aprons with appliqués of cupcakes on the bib, leather sandals, pottery and more pottery, gemstones, bath products, woodcrafts, and decorative pieces in blown glass, and past the beer tent, the rain room (a tent whose walls somehow emit a fine, cooling mist of water), and a rock-climbing wall.

But where's the garlic?

In the nick of time the Garlic Information Center appears. A nice young woman behind the counter tells me there are no talks or seminars but there is a garlic-braiding class and a garlic-topping contest. Unfortunately, I've just missed both for the day. However, if I'd like one, I could have a free garlic-growing kit . . .

"Or," she points across the field, "you could head on over to the Christopher Ranch booth. They have lots of garlic for sale."

At the booth I ask what varieties they have, and does one of them happen to be a French pink garlic? "Never heard of pink garlic," says the young man. "I've seen purple-skinned and purple-striped, even brownish garlic, but not pink. This nice big white one here is the only one we have. It's what we grow at Christopher Ranch." He points to a bin of pearly white bulbs with many cloves bulging under their glistening, pristine skin. Every year Christopher Ranch, the largest grower of garlic in North America and the pride of Gilroy, donates hundreds of pounds of the Artichoke cultivar 'California Early' to be cooked at Gourmet Alley and in the festival's demonstrations and competitions. It's being sold as single bulbs, in bags, or in braids. 'California Early' and 'California Late,' which isn't ready for market yet, are the mainstay of the California garlic industry, with 'Early' most often used for processing. I buy two huge bulbs for a start.

The afternoon wears on. The sun beats down, and suddenly I'm depleted, my throat dry. Where is Suzy? Samples of garlic ice cream, courtesy of Gilroy Foods, are available at a small booth not too far from the crowded beer garden, but the lineup snakes halfway across the field. Maybe tomorrow. My feet hurt. I wander more, find a big booth selling plastic cups of creamy frozen lemonade, buy one, and sink gratefully onto another straw bale in a cooling grove of redwood trees. This bale is offered by a young man who jumps to his feet as I draw near and says, "Ma'am? Sit here." Man, was I looking that bad? I can't swallow the frozen lemonade and have to let it melt in my mouth and slide down my throat.

Fate intervenes with a sign. I glance up and see it straight ahead of me: "Cook-Off Stage." I know in an instant that is where I should be.

And that's where I happily spend the rest of the weekend.

---

*After you eat a lot of garlic you just kind of feel like
you are floating, you feel ultra-confident, you feel capable of
going out and whipping your weight in wildcats.*
MICHAEL GOODWIN, food and film writer,
in *Garlic Is as Good as Ten Mothers*

THE COOK-OFF Stage is where it's happening, for this festival is really all about food, food with lots of garlic. All around me a happy throng of food lovers watch the chopping and sautéing taking place on the vast stage in event after event. My eyes are glued to the goings-on too. A handful of luxe-looking cooking stations with ovens, gas cooktops, and sinks with hot water are set up for the chefs, professional and amateur, who are taking part. A table on one side of the stage, where the judges taste and exclaim—usually into a microphone—is nicely set with good china.

Volunteer cooking assistants mill about. TV crews carefully pick their way through the proceedings, filming the sweating chefs in close-up and medium frame, while their assistants carefully keep the cables out of the way. Close-ups are displayed on two immense screens on either side of the stage, food porn for us to slaver over. A sunscreen over the stage and the bleachers keeps the rest of us cool and comfortable—and cuts glare for the TV cameras.

It's Food Network outdoors, live, with no commercials. The shows go on all day without a break. Everyone is having fun—the important thing at the Gilroy Garlic Festival—and I am too.

From the beginning, the festival has had a sixth sense for publicity. In 1979 the first festival played a role in Les Blank's garlic-giddy documentary *Garlic Is as Good as Ten Mothers*. It features one of the three founders, Val Filice, who died in 2007. A second founder, Rudy Melone, died in 1998. The third founder, Don Christopher, happens to sit down beside me in the front row of the bleachers as I'm settling in for the rest of the afternoon.

"Aren't you Don Christopher?" I ask. "I saw your picture on the program—you're just the fellow I'd like to talk to." He looks at me a little like I'm a door-to-door salesman who's just shown up at dinnertime, but he agrees to chat a while. "Val had a personality and presence like no one else," he says. "He got the cooperation of everyone." Don credits Rudy with coming up with the idea for the festival. Rudy was convinced Gilroy was the true garlic capital of the world in spite of a claim made by Arleux, France, which was drawing seventy thousand people to its annual festival in the 1970s. All Gilroy had to do was have a bigger festival to prove it, Rudy said, and it's been doing that every year since.

As for himself, Don says he's just a farmer at heart, born on a prune farm near Gilroy with a love of the earth in his genes. But he grew up with a strong entrepreneurial streak. As a lad of twenty-two he bought land and started Christopher Ranch to grow garlic. One might say that organizing a garlic festival with his buddies once he got established didn't hurt his business, but both Christopher Ranch and the festival have done a lot for Gilroy.

Christopher Ranch harvests 65 million pounds (30 million kilos) of garlic a year in eight fields around Gilroy as well as on leased land in Monterey County and the San Joaquin Valley. "We supply California garlic to the whole country, including parts of Canada, every day of the year," Don says. "We even borrowed something from the apple guys: we built special cold-storage facilities where we take all the oxygen out and put the garlic to sleep till we need it."

Don looks more than a little grim when I mention Chinese garlic. "A few years ago China brought garlic into the United States below cost and took over a whole lot of the market," he says. "In fact, it took over nearly the whole world, including Canada. We had to cut our acreage down to about 55 percent." But then the flow started to slow down. With next to no money coming into their pockets, Don says, Chinese farmers got wise and quit growing garlic in favor of other vegetables. "We didn't know that had happened till suddenly the Chinese price went up to nearly match ours."

But Don hadn't let the opportunities of cheap Chinese garlic slip through his fingers. "I bought a lot of it and sold it at a profit," he says.

"You did? No kidding," I respond. Now there's bold entrepreneurial spirit.

"Yes, I did. And we sold it rapidly. Everyone was going crazy about the situation, but I figured if I could make a little money on it while others wept, why not?"

"You didn't sell it as your own garlic, did you?" I ask, a little worried about Don's scruples.

"I wouldn't do *that!*" He looks surprised that I would even suggest such a thing. "We wouldn't compete with ourselves. We often buy and sell garlic from other countries if we think we're going to be short or if we have too much. We sold it as Chinese garlic to people who were already buying Chinese garlic. So I made money on it, and I had a lot of fun, too."

Don isn't exactly a garlic lover himself. He eats it maybe three times a week, slivered and inserted into the meat he barbecues. "I prefer to grow it," he says. "I love seeing those green tips coming up in spring when everything else is going into the ground. But what I like the best is marketing it. It's exciting. I like dealing with buyers and agreeing on a price, I like packing it and shipping it. And I like developing products, like the green garlic we package for garnish and the like. You harvest it when it's eight to twelve weeks along. Its stalks are tender and mild..."

He looks over my shoulder and waves at his little granddaughter. "She's looking for me," he says. He's had enough chat and is clearly itching to get moving. That's okay—I've had a revealing glimpse of some of the energy that's made the Gilroy Garlic Festival so successful all these years.

The growing and processing of garlic
will move to China. There's nothing to stop it.
CAO MENGHUI, Jinan Yipin Corp. Ltd.,
garlic producer and exporter, Shandong, China

NEARLY THE whole world, not just Don Christopher, is angry about Chinese garlic and the way it's been marketed and exported—or dumped, to be blunt. And some countries aren't going to take it anymore. They've been fighting back with huge tariffs or fines, plus jail sentences for garlic smuggling. Yes, cheap Chinese garlic is such a prized commodity in some places that it's smuggled across borders disguised as onions or other produce. But the big issue in North America over the past decade has been dumping, and it's forced many garlic growers to reduce production, like Don Christopher, or to go out of business entirely.

In the United States, the first wave of Chinese garlic appeared in the mid-1990s, at half the cost of California garlic. The Chinese were found to be selling it at less than their cost—which, given their workers' subsistence wages plus the inexpensive containers used to ship goods, is ridiculously low to begin with. The United States levied a hefty 377 percent tariff on the garlic, the highest imposed on any product crossing its borders. It slowed down imports for a few years, but the Chinese claimed they weren't dumping and filed for a review of the charges, leading to a lengthy hearing.

Then a loophole in the regulations was discovered, and Chinese garlic began to make its way back into California and other American ports. Imports increased tenfold in three years in the mid-2000s, to 86 million pounds (39 million kilos) by 2005, 5 million pounds (2.3 million kilos) more garlic than was grown in California and up from a meager 365,000 pounds (166,000 kilos) in 2000. The industry was shrinking in California: from 1999 to 2004, the number of acres devoted to growing garlic dropped from 40,000 to 26,000 (from 16,000 to 10,000 hectares), and some growers said they were making no profit at all.

Lawyers for the American garlic industry defending the tariff argued that the Chinese wanted to corner the U.S. market, and the Chinese were accused of using fraudulent schemes to avoid paying customs duties, such as shipping through countries like Vietnam and Japan and falsifying the true country of origin. "The system is not set up to deal with the degree of creativity the Chinese bring to the market," one lawyer for the California producers told a reporter for SFGate.com.

In Canada, the situation was, and is, similar. "In 2001, China began dumping garlic on the Ontario market for about 40 cents a pound [88 cents a kilo] wholesale. A grower here needed $1.50 to make it viable," says Mark Wales, president of the Garlic Growers Association of Ontario. "I call that predatory dumping." He, too, thinks the Chinese want to take over the garlic industry.

Canadian garlic had its start as an industry in the late 1980s, when farmers planted garlic and ginseng as alternatives to the once-lucrative tobacco crops. It takes a few years to establish a good supply of garlic because it's grown not from seed, as are other vegetables, but from the six to twelve cloves each plant produces, resulting in six to twelve plants—a lot less than the hundreds of plants possible from the seeds of a beet or a carrot. It takes years for a garlic crop to become large enough to supply the market. By 2000, 3,500 to 4,000 acres (1,400 to 1,600 hectares) of garlic were being grown commercially in Ontario (which grows 95 percent of Canada's garlic). Then the Chinese invaded. Canadian garlic wasn't worth the cost of harvesting.

"The crop size dropped to about 400 acres in one season," Mark says. Within two years it was down to 200, or about 80 hectares. "Our association was successful in getting a five-year tariff of about 80 cents a pound [$1.75 a kilo] levied on the garlic. That brought the Chinese wholesale price up to about $1.25, the same as garlic from Mexico. There was no garlic from China anymore, but all of a sudden 11 million kilos"—24 million pounds—"the same as had come from China, was coming in from Pakistan and the Philippines, countries that had never shipped garlic to Canada before." Although the invoices said the products were from those countries, in many cases the original labels were still on the box: "Product of China."

The tariff expired in 2007, and it wasn't renewed, at least in part because the garlic growers felt the government hadn't been vigilant in enforcing the rules when it was obvious that the Pakistani and Filipino garlic originated in China. The shame of it is that domestic garlic was on the brink of commercial success in 2001. Warren Ham, director of anti-dumping for the Garlic Growers Association of Ontario and a grower himself, says the industry was robust enough to supply all the garlic the market needed; it might even have built a climate-controlled warehouse, like the one at Christopher Ranch, so that supplies could be available nearly year-round.

"But it's not as if we can't get back there again," he says. "We have a choice: we could put our garlic back in the ground and wrap up production for five years down the road till we can supply bigger crops." Or garlic could continue to be what it's become: a cottage industry, marketed at fairs and farmers' markets and via mail order. But if growers decide to invest in the future by propagating their crops of garlic for a few years, they need to find another way to earn enough income to support their families in the meantime.

Like most consumers, I had little idea of the effect Chinese garlic had had on growers; I was more consumed by the effect it had on me. How many times have I exchanged complaints with fellow shoppers over bins of those Asian bulbs, deploring the small size that makes the tiny inner cloves hardly worth the effort it takes to peel them, or the little green shoots that mean the garlic is past its prime, or the squishy feeling under the papery skin that means it's advanced to the point of death? But the garlic effect goes further than the grocery store and mild complaints between shoppers, and it's arguably bigger than the problems American and Canadian growers are experiencing. It's also started trade wars and has caused political conflict in other countries.

In Thailand in 2008 the price of garlic dropped from 40 baht to about 17 baht per kilo (from 60 cents to 25 cents per pound)— less than it cost to grow it—and created hardship for many less-than-affluent growers. The culprit was Chinese garlic, huge amounts of which were allowed into the country under a trade agreement. The government's solution was to encourage the cultivation of potatoes, which were relatively inexpensive to grow. But where were they to be sold? Potatoes aren't a big part of the Thai diet, and what market there was demanded only perfectly uniform potatoes in pristine condition.

Farmers protested. Garlic became part of an overall political issue as garlic growers joined truck drivers, rice farmers, and fishermen, all wanting assistance in fighting inflation. Samak Sundaravej, who was prime minister of Thailand for a few months in 2008 and considered himself a gourmand (he was known for his pork marinated in Coca-Cola), tried to alleviate the garlic situation. In one of his Sunday addresses to the country he praised the virtues of the beautifully flavorful and much stronger Thai garlic and urged citizens to use it. But the prime minister spoke out of both sides of his mouth. At about the same time an existing highway through Laos from Kunming, China, to Bangkok was being refurbished to cut the driving time of trucks bringing garlic and other fruits and vegetables from China to Thailand.

In Korea, a trade war over garlic erupted in 2000. Koreans were angry about cheap Chinese garlic, so a 315 percent tariff was slapped on it. China thought that was unfair, so it declared a ban on Korea's mobile phones and polyethylene products. The dispute seems one-sided, however, since Korea's banned products amounted to about US$413 million, whereas the garlic from China was worth about US$15 million.

Does *anyone* like Chinese garlic?

Well, smugglers do. It's cheap, and if you can find a way to avoid the customs duties levied by many countries, you might make a fortune. Then again, you might get caught.

The Calcutta *Telegraph* reported that in late January 2011, in a midnight operation, more than 11,000 pounds (5,000 kilos) of Chinese garlic were seized in and around the railway station in Raxaul, India. It had been brought over the border by women and children, presumably because they would arouse less suspicion than a group of men. The previous December, nearly one hundred sacks were seized in the same place. The garlic came from Nepal, where it costs half what it does in India.

In Poland in January 2011, European Union customs police seized six shipping containers containing garlic disguised as onions, which are taxed at a lower rate. The garlic had come from China via Rotterdam and wasn't the first shipment to be caught.

In 2009, a similar quantity of Chinese garlic had been smuggled into the European Union via Norway, which exempts garlic from customs duties, by an international group of smugglers. The garlic was worth an estimated €1.5 million in customs duties to the European countries it was surreptitiously headed for. The smuggling had gone on for some time, apparently, and the European Anti-Fraud Office launched an investigation in May 2010. A month later a truck carrying a full load of garlic was stopped.

But let's be honest here. The smugglers aren't the only ones who like Chinese garlic. North American grocery chains like it, too, even if most of their customers don't. But who can blame them? Chinese garlic is cheap, plentiful, and always available. Of course it's plentiful—China grows 75 percent of the world's garlic.

• WHERE GARLIC GROWS •

In 2008, the Food and Agricultural Organization of the United Nations came up with a list of the top ten garlic producers in the world. Figures are in tonnes.

China	12,088,000
India	645,000
South Korea	325,000
Egypt	258,608
Russia	254,000
United States	221,810
Spain	142,400
Argentina	140,000
Myanmar	128,000
Ukraine	125,000

THE PROBLEM for small growers—and few garlic-growing operations on this continent are big—is that they can't guarantee a large supply of garlic year-round, which is what big chains want. They may not even be able to supply a large enough amount from August to December, when garlic is in season, having been harvested in late July or August and stored under the usual conditions until winter. That's where a climate-controlled storage building would be valuable. But first, as Warren Ham says, growers—in Ontario especially, where most of Canada's garlic is grown—have to get back to where they were in 2001 and produce enough garlic to satisfy the demands of the big chains.

One wonders why the big chains can't buy small quantities of produce like garlic and tomatoes from local producers instead of bombarding us with imports in our bountiful harvest season. So I was heartened to see Galen Weston, executive chairman of Loblaw Companies Limited (which owns just over a thousand stores and franchises across Canada, including the namesake stores, No Frills, Superstore, Fortinos, Zehrs, and more), advertising the company's initiative to buy local wherever possible. Would that include garlic? I wondered. How lovely if we could find some really good local bulbs in the grocery bins, maybe an 'Ontario Giant,' a Rocambole, or the popular 'Music,' a Porcelain brought to Ontario from Italy in the 1980s. So I called head office and asked to speak to the vp of produce procurement about his garlic plans and his take on the Chinese garlic situation. I didn't get past the public relations department, which intervened and asked me to submit a list of questions. After a few days, I got the following reply: "Upon further review, we believe this is an industry related subject and feel you would be better suited following up with the Retail Council of Canada."

China doesn't even grow the many varieties now available in most of the rest of the world. "We have two kinds—softneck and hardneck," says John Huang, North American representative for Pretty Garlic, one of the biggest importers of Asian garlic to this continent. "We don't use the other classifications other countries do. Softneck is what we sell, in pure white and regular white, which has a bit of a purple stripe on the skin."

As Don Christopher and others have said, there was a period when the supply of garlic dwindled in China and the price went up. In 2009 it nearly quadrupled, making garlic one of the country's best assets that year. Why? As in any other country and with any agricultural product, prices are dependent on many influences—floods and frost, supply and demand, and, in China, even influenza epidemics. Yes, the flu: economists at Morgan Stanley, an international financial adviser, theorized the trigger for the price increase might have been the H1N1 virus and the faith the Chinese have in garlic's ability to ward off disease. A story in the *China Daily* bolstered this argument: it reported that a high school in Hangzhou, a city in eastern China, had bought enough garlic for all its students to eat every day at lunch so that they would stay healthy. John Huang says garlic's medicinal properties affected its price in the beginning, but the weak global economy was likely a stronger influence. The garlic market suffered along with other markets, and when farmers began to receive less for their garlic, they started to plant less—about 50 percent less, in fact. Garlic became a valuable commodity for investment and the price went up. Stories abound about people who bought garlic, stored it, and waited for the price to climb higher. One story claims a young man in his early twenties borrowed money provided to the banks by the government to keep the economy going, bought a load of garlic, flipped it when the price went up, and used the proceeds to buy a Toyota.

"It's true: in 2009 and 2010 speculators were successful in controlling the market," says John Huang. "They bought garlic, held it back, and forced prices higher as supplies became limited."

But then the expected happened: farmers planted more garlic because the price looked good. "More garlic, lower prices," John says. "The 2011 crop is 30 percent more than 2010's. Prices are dropping, dropping, dropping."

My next-door neighbor's father-in-law grows vegetables in the Holland Marsh region north of Toronto, the vegetable basket of the province, and sells them at the Ontario Food Terminal in Toronto. Let's put that in the past tense—he used to grow them. In an over-the-fence conversation one day he tells my husband he's switched from veggies to herbs. "I can't compete with the price of Chinese imports," he says.

In the United States, the garlic situation has changed slightly. Bill Christopher, Don's son and a partner in the family company, says consumers and food distributors have become much more concerned about where their food is coming from and care more about buying local produce. "Food safety and traceability of food sources are important," he says. "China's smaller-than-usual crop enabled U.S. suppliers to retake some markets and explain the benefits of locally grown produce."

But what's next, now that China once again has a large crop to export?

"I think 2012 will be an interesting year," he says.

Garlic is my salt and pepper.

MARGEE BERRY, first-prize winner, Great Garlic Cook-Off

I HAVE a special reason for being on time for Saturday's Great Garlic Cook-Off: I'd entered a recipe in the contest months before and sometimes, in the moments before falling asleep, I'd fantasized about preparing the dish onstage and then modestly accepting a prize. Not necessarily first—second or third would do. Even being among the eight finalists would be grand.

My recipe didn't even make the first cut. It's a simple dish of steamed rapini sautéed in olive oil and chopped garlic (the rules require no less than 3 teaspoons, or 15 mL), served over soft garlic-and-basil polenta, and topped with a poached egg, with garlic-laced salsa fresca on the side. It's one of my favorite breakfasts, one I came up with when I had some leftover rapini and polenta in the fridge, and I thought it was an easy but good-tasting recipe the judges might like. Once I see what the eight finalists—who'd been selected from hundreds of entries—are cooking up there on the stage, and what seasoned contest participants they are, I realize what I'd been up against. Their recipes are much more creative than mine. While the judges are tallying their results (and because I'd managed to wangle a media badge that allowed me on the Cook-Off Stage), I have a taste of Penny Malcolm's Roasted Garlic, Blueberry, and Pear Cobbler with Garlic-Pecan Brickle Cream. "This is amazing," I say as the flavors explode in my mouth. It's sweet and savory, smooth and crunchy. And the subtle taste of garlic fits right in. Penny grins.

"I also entered a Brie pecan pie with garlic, but it didn't make it to the finals, so don't feel bad about yours," she says. She's come here from Americus, Georgia, to prepare her cobbler on stage. "This is the third time I've entered and the first time I made it to the finals. But unlike some of the other competitions I've been in, this one is pretty informal, so it's easier."

"The others?" I exclaim. "How many do you enter?"

"About twenty-four a year," she says matter-of-factly.

"How many have you won?"

"Twelve. It can rule your life after a while."

Penny's amazing cobbler doesn't win. Margee Berry's Warm-Weather Watermelon Crabmeat-Kissed South Seas Soup takes first place. Margee's no stranger to the Gilroy contest either. "I won third prize here about nine years ago, then second six years ago," she says. She came from Trout Lake, Washington, the day before to shop for ingredients, as did the other contestants, who are expected to supply everything except the garlic. "Once you win you have to wait three years to enter again. But I figured I had a pattern going and this time I was sure to take first."

Her cool soup has a contemporary combination of flavors perfect for a hot summer day. At first it's sweet, then minty. The garlic appears and then backs off and you taste the ginger, the hot chilies and lemongrass. The flavors remain separate—just the way food is in Thailand.

Leslie Shearer's Potentially Pretentious Pork Tenderloin with Garlic Five Ways takes second place. "You should have won first just for the name," I say to her. Her big laugh fills the space between us. "It's really poking a bit of fun at over-engineered restaurant food with complicated names," she says. "I also figured it wouldn't hurt to have a catchy name to make the judges take notice."

They take notice—they smack their lips over Leslie's pork. "That first taste of the garlic chip sealed it for me," enthuses one. "Then the creamy goat cheese played off the pork and the tanginess and sweetness of the sauce."

"The texture of the grit cakes was so sensual," rhapsodizes another. "It's the kind of food they ate in that movie *Tom Jones*. Fabulous treatment of garlic."

The recipe contains four heads of roasted garlic and six cloves of sliced fried garlic, grits cooked in garlic-infused water, garlic powder, four cloves of minced garlic for roasting the pork, and... hmm, I guess that's five ways. Also included: softened goat cheese, arugula tossed in the garlic-roasting oil, a reduction of balsamic vinegar and fig preserves, and the roasted pork, of course. "See what I mean?" says Leslie. "It's definitely potentially pretentious."

Suzy shows up waving a foot-long grilled and garlicky, beautifully buttery cob of corn.

"This is so delicious," she calls. "Let's go eat!"

And so we share more garlic-laden foods: barbecued pork on a bun, a large steamed artichoke filled with shrimp and crab Louis, and Cajun crawdads. What's a festival without lots of food? Then we sample some local wine in the big and busy Rotary International tent and totter back to our bed-and-breakfast for a nap.

I wouldn't go to Baskin-Robbins for it.
Overheard in the lineup for garlic ice cream

THE FIRST place I head Sunday morning is the lineup for garlic ice cream. There are about a dozen people waiting, and I have my little cone in my hand in no time. I lick. First it tasted like plain vanilla, then I get garlic on the back of my tongue, and it expands as the ice cream melts down my throat. Do I sound like a wine columnist? But when it comes down to it, it's ice cream with a hint of garlic. I expect there's no market for it beyond the festival.

I spend the rest of the day at the Garlic Showdown, where four professional chefs compete for a $5,000 prize, creating dishes on the spot with garlic and a mystery ingredient to be revealed when the contest begins. Very *Iron Chef*. The emcee is Fabio Viviani, successful West Coast restaurateur, cookbook author, and *Top Chef*'s Season 5 Fan Favorite (and winner of $10,000 for the distinction). He falls into his role right away, striding the stage like Mick Jagger, cracking jokes, promoting products, and engaging in crowd-pleasing hijinks while keeping track of the chefs' progress for the audience.

This year's special ingredient is mushrooms, and each chef is given a box of several varieties. They have an hour to prepare and present two dishes—after all, they are professionals—and most of them outdo themselves and come up with several. Ryan Scott, the defending champion, wins again. He owns Ryan Scott 2 Go catering in San Francisco, and even at his tender age (he's in his mid-thirties) he'd been head chef at a couple of well-known Bay Area restaurants before opening his business. His winning recipe is in three parts: Perplexed Portobello Steak with Mushroom Purée and Mushroom Crudo. *P* alliterations seem to be in the air this weekend. "I named it that because the mushrooms are seared like a steak, so I figured they weren't sure of their identities," jokes Ryan. The mushrooms were plated on the garlic-mushroom purée and topped with mushroom jus from the pan and then mushroom crudo.

It's well after two on the last day of the festival, and after watching the preparation of such elegant food and being denied even a mouthful, Suzy and I are ravenous. A Ryan Scott 2 Go booth is conveniently located directly across the field, and we hotfoot it over there with half the audience. We line up for sweet and succulent pulled pork and crisp coleslaw on a bun, but the garlic sweet-potato fries are sold out. It's probably a good thing. By the time we've finished the pork we need to do a brisk round of the grounds and some final shopping to shake it down.

"Did you have a good time?" says the man at the media tent as we're leaving.

"It was fabulous. I'm overwhelmed," I say. "I don't know how you do it."

"I didn't think I could have so much fun at a garlic festival," says Suzy. "And for three whole days."

And we both mean every mouthwatering word of it.

A day without garlic is a day without sunshine.
Sign outside a greengrocer in Lautrec, France

ON THE first day of our visit to Lautrec, Chris and I spot the pink garlic as soon as we walk past a little food shop on the narrow and cobblestoned Rue du Mercadial, just inside the village gate. Tightly tied bunches of perfectly round and uniformly plump garlic bulbs nestle together in a bin, glistening in a slanted ray of sunlight like pink satin. They look polished. I study them for a few moments before picking up a bunch, almost afraid to break the spell. I've come a long way to find this garlic.

I want to rip off the skin right away to see if the cloves inside are pink, but I resist the urge. The one-pound (450-gram) bunches, called *manouilles,* of nine identical bulbs sell for seven euros in village shops and at Lautrec's Friday morning market. In the nearby city of Castres they're nine or ten euros, and at Fauchon in

Paris, twenty euros. In London they cost even more. It's expensive garlic, and it's important to Lautrec. Around the village more land is devoted to growing sunflowers than to garlic, but they don't bring in as many euros as pink garlic. Pink garlic is grown on about 20 percent of the land but represents about 80 percent of the local agricultural economy.

The Fête de l'Ail Rose is the next day, and the villagers are preparing in a restrained French way. A few signs announce the one-day event and give locations for the judging of the garlic art (no kidding—sculptures and tableaus are made from every part of the plant, and some of them are worthy of display in your living room) and for the *fabounade,* the evening banquet, where the big cassoulet will be served after the ceremonial procession led by the Brotherhood of Pink Garlic. But no booths or tents are being set up—that will start before dawn on festival day. And there's not a sign of preparations for the famous pink garlic soup, the festival's main attraction, which brings people from miles around. It will be served to hundreds in the Place Centrale at noon sharp.

Although the scent of garlic is absent, the walled village of Lautrec (population under two thousand, in southwest France, about 53 miles, or 85 kilometers, from Toulouse) is rich with history, from its thirteenth-century corbelled and half-timbered houses to the faintly touristy clog maker's workshop, the restored 1688 windmill, and the incredible trompe l'oeil frescoes in the Collegiate Church of Saint Rémy. They were painted about 1850 and rival the frescoes in many more prosperous European churches. The village even boasts a couple of *parterres de broderie* attributed to the great André Le Nôtre, who designed gardens at Versailles, Vaux-le-Vicomte, and Chantilly for Louis XIV.

By eating the good soup made with our garlic.
You will live as long as our land has.
Ail! Ail! Ail!
Song of the Brotherhood of Pink Garlic

A cross near the top of the hill that dominates Lautrec marks the site of the original home—or castle—of the viscounts of Toulouse and Lautrec, who founded the village about AD 1000. Yes, the late-nineteenth-century painter and printmaker Henri de Toulouse-Lautrec came by his name honestly: he was a descendant of the dynasty that built this little village, although he was born in Albi, an equally historic city about 18 miles (30 kilometers) distant. The hill was a well-chosen site for the family headquarters: from its height the countryside could be watched, and the village grew to need protection. The fertile soil made it prosperous agriculturally, as did an industry that produced a distinctive robin's-egg-blue dye from the dried leaves of *Isalis tinctoria* (a member of the mustard family commonly called woad); like garlic today, the dye was a staple of the economics of the area before the days of indigo, and the color is seen on doors and shutters throughout Lautrec. Lautrec was also vulnerable because it was a Catholic fief in a predominantly non-Catholic area, and by 1338 it had become a fortress protected by a wall 4,000 feet (1,200 meters) long. A good portion of the ramparts and one of the original eight gates—the Porte de la Caussade, through which Chris and I entered—remain today. So does the hill, now castle-less but a lovely spot for contemplation, as we discover, shaded and grassy and outfitted with benches from which you can enjoy the cooling breeze and gaze out at the Lacaune

Hills, the Black Mountains, and the plain of Castres. On a clear day you can see the Pyrenees in the distance.

IT'S NINE-THIRTY on Friday, the morning of the festival, and a hundred men and women resplendent in ceremonial robes are marching behind a brass band down Rue du Mercadial, singing the ode to pink garlic with unbridled enthusiasm—in French, of course, and to the tune of an old children's song. Pauline Danigo, a young student of languages, has offered to help the French-challenged Canadian through the day, and she translates it for me.

The marchers, looking very serious and followed by dozens of festivalgoers, turn the corner where Pauline and I are standing—Chris is off taking pictures—and carefully pick their way down the steep, cobbled street to the *théâtre de plein air*, a stone amphitheater built over the subterranean silos where grain was stored in the Middle Ages. Proudly leading the pack are the men and women of the brotherhood, the Confrérie de l'Ail Rose, wearing deep green cloaks with puffy white sleeves and white straw fedoras. The brotherhoods that follow—the Confrérie de la Poule Farcie and the Confrérie de la Poule au Pot et Fromage de Barousse; the Confrérie de l'Omelette Géante and the *confréries* of tomatoes, mushrooms, cherries, truffles, and du Puy lentils; the Académie du Châteaubriant, supporters of the wines of Toulouse and Gaillac; and for some reason the brotherhood of stonecutters—are attired in embroidered satin and velvet like archbishops and cardinals on their way to an ordination. The bright orange velvet cloaks with feathery green collars worn by the carrots of Blagnac are crowd-pleasers, and everyone claps as they go by. Then they cheer for a plump white-haired gentleman with the Ordre de la Dive Bouteille de Gaillac, who rather dangerously jives down the steep street, grinning and loving the attention.

The French love their food and drink. There are more than six hundred *confréries* in twenty-six regions of the country, and many have been around since medieval times. The pink garlic brotherhood is a new kid in the group—it was organized in 2000. Each *confrérie* worships at the altar of its own gastronomic idol, celebrating and promoting it. "They're pretty social groups, actually," says Pauline, whose grandmother is a grower and has been a member of the garlic brotherhood since it began. "They're always meeting and eating. I think they just like one another's company."

The *confréries* take their places on the stone seats of the little amphitheater, and the onlookers, including me, hang over the low wall or stand around in any available space. The speeches begin. "They're saying how great it is to be together here today and that they'll be bringing into the garlic brotherhood some new members from other groups, like the carrots, the omelettes, the Toulouse wine, the stonecutters, and the eel people—they're from near Perpignan, on the Mediterranean," Pauline says. There's an eruption of laughter. "They like to tell funny anecdotes about each other, too."

The inductees come up to the stage one by one, accompanied by a pink garlic brother or sister who stands behind and places a green cloak over each new member's shoulders. "Those are the sponsors—they call them godmothers or godfathers," Pauline says.

• WHAT'S IN A LABEL? •

Pink garlic was grown informally around Lautrec until 1959, when several young producers formed the Syndicat de Défense du Label Ail Rose de Lautrec to improve growing and marketing practices. In 1966 the garlic was awarded the Label Rouge, which officially identifies quality and is an award of prestige in France. About 185 growers and three packaging houses are now part of the Syndicat de Défense du Label Rouge et de l'IGP Ail Rose de Lautrec, growing garlic in the southwestern department of Tarn. Yield hovers between 660 and 770 tons (600 to 700 tonnes) annually.

In 1996 pink garlic received an IGP, the Indication Géographique Protégée, a European label that certifies that agricultural products have been grown in a specified area in the framework of IGP-PGI rules and have been checked by the awarding body.

A long wooden staff bound at one end with sixteen pink garlic heads is handed to the Grand Chancellor, who solemnly touches both shoulders of the inductees and says a few words we can't hear. Large bibs are tied around the new members' necks.

"Initiation," whispers Pauline, finger to her lips. It's a solemn moment. A steaming pot is brought to the stage. "They have to eat a bowl of the pink garlic soup."

The brotherhood bursts into song as the inductees carefully sip: *"En mangeant la bonne soupe faite avec notre ail, vous vivrez comme naguère aussi vieux que notre terre. Ail! Ail! Ail!"*

"But why do they sound like they're pigs squealing at the end of the song?" I whisper back. "Are they implying the garlic stings your tongue?"

Pauline laughs. "It's a French play on words," she explains. "*Ail* means garlic but it's pronounced like *aïe*, like when you say 'Ouch!' Repeating it three times is a custom here. It doesn't mean anything. It's just there because it sounds good."

I look blank. "I guess it's a French thing," says Pauline.

When the ceremony is over we find a bench and Pauline goes to look for her grandmother. Jacqueline Barthe joins us, removes her white fedora and fans her face. It might be hot, but she is an official and her cloak has to stay put for the ceremonial opening of the grand soup tasting in an hour. She pats her white bob and waits for me to say something. "She understands English pretty well, but she asked me to translate her answers," Pauline says.

"Um, so how much garlic do you grow?" I begin. She's trying to retire, she says, so she cut her acreage in half a couple of years ago, to 2.5 acres (1 hectare). "That's four thousand kilos of garlic," close to nine thousand pounds, she says.

"IS IT hard to meet all the requirements of the Syndicat? I understand the regulations are pretty tough."

"If the weather is bad and it affects your garlic, they don't penalize you. But if it's you who's made the mistake, you have two chances. The first year, a warning. The second year, *fini!*" She slaps her knee vehemently.

She was warned once for a small infraction that had nothing to do with the quality of the garlic: she'd left the lot number off her trays.

"And that was all?" I say in disbelief.

"The records must be perfect." Madame Barthe looks stern. "There are rules for the Label Rouge and the IGP"—the Indication Géographique Protégée, or Protected Geographical Indication, a legal designation that protects the names of regional foods in much the same way as the appellation system controls wines. "Pink garlic is special, and we must keep it that way."

"But what makes it such a special garlic?" I ask.

She turns directly to me. Her eyes flash.

"*C'est le terroir!*" she says emphatically. The chalky clay soil, dry and hard, the sun, and the right amount of rain give it the mellow taste and good storage qualities. There is only a small area with the right conditions for growing perfect pink garlic. Lautrec may seem like a quaint French village immersed in history, and its festival may not be big and showy, but its garlic growers know a thing or two about marketing and protecting their unique product. Chinese garlic wouldn't dare compete with Ail Rose, not here, and not in Paris or London, either.

"Um, do you like to eat garlic yourself?" I ask Madame Barthe, feeling chastened.

"Ah, *comme ci, comme ça*," she says, waving her hand. "I don't put it in everything."

"But she makes a really delicious garlic pie," says Pauline. "The whole family adores it. It gave her the idea to start a garlic pie contest at the festival."

"I like the garlic soup best," Madame Barthe says. "This year it won a new designation for Lautrec—Site Remarquable du Goût, which the state awards to a place that offers extra-special food or drink." She looks pleased and proud but suggests we should hurry along to the Place Centrale if we want to watch the soup making. "It will be ready to eat soon," she says.

Place Centrale is jammed with hundreds of people pressing up against a metal barrier that keeps them away from the cooking area, which is under the wooden loggia of the beautifully restored brick market building. Although they're dressed in contemporary gear and are waiting patiently, I suddenly have an image of peasants outside Louis XVI's palace clamoring for bread. Or would that be cake?

"The cooking area is also the VIP area," says Pauline. "My grandmother said we can go in there to watch and get our soup."

And watch we do, Chris, Pauline, and I, while sniffing the intoxicating aroma of hundreds, perhaps thousands, of cloves of pink garlic making themselves into an ambrosial soup. Time moves backward, and I relive the moment decades ago when Joe and I walked into Luca's Italian restaurant and I met garlic nose-on for the first time. Six cauldrons are being stirred over propane burners, a thousand liters of garlic soup, about 250 gallons. Will everyone waiting go away happy, a bowl of soup in hand, or might there be a revolution?

One woman is clearly in charge, and she has twenty assistants. They started at eight that morning, filling the cauldrons with water and bringing it to the boil. Once the water reached the right temperature, hundreds of cloves of finely chopped pink garlic were added. I watch mustard and huge cans of mayonnaise go in, then broken pieces of vermicelli. Young men with dependable muscles constantly stir the mixture to keep it smooth. And the boss lady appears every so often to dip her ladle in and taste. Stirring and tasting, stirring and tasting. We mill about sipping

• SMALL BUT MIGHTY •

The one-day Fête de l'Ail Rose de Lautrec began in 1970 and always takes place the first Friday in August. It attracts close to ten thousand people, though arriving at that figure is an inexact science, because admission is not charged. The organizers do informal head counts in the square a couple of times during the day, especially when the garlic soup is being served and the biggest crowd is in attendance.

Sixty or seventy volunteers are involved, and the expense budget is about £25,000. Promoting pink garlic and Lautrec is the festival's main goal, but each year it donates about £400 to a charitable association, usually for disabled children.

white wine with the VIPs and a small television crew. Outside the barrier, the crowd remains patient. Some of the older people sit in rows of chairs set up for the soup event. "People come early and stand in the square for hours," says Pauline.

The soup is worth the wait. It's strong, sweet, smooth, and simple all at once, with "strong" being the operative word. It tastes overwhelmingly of garlic, but mellow garlic. The vermicelli makes a perfect balance of texture. "This is the best soup I've ever tasted," says Chris. As we slurp our soup the rest is being ladled into plastic bowls and passed out to the first row pressing against the barrier, along with a glass of wine for each. How do people manage to turn and carry the hot soup and cold wine back through the crowd behind them without spilling? The French are more adept than me.

Meanwhile, the garlic pies are arriving at the judging center across the square, carried in by husbands or the bakers themselves in boxes or on trays covered with plastic wrap held up by toothpicks to protect the filling. There are fourteen entries by deadline time. I crane my neck through a three-deep row of onlookers to watch as the pies are gently unwrapped, given numbers, and placed in a refrigerated glass case. To a pie they'd been baked in those scalloped French tarte pans with removable bottoms, a lovely concept fraught with the specter of broken pastry and a ruined pie when you try to slide it off the bottom. These pies slide off perfectly intact. Is it the skill of the unpacker or the perfect texture of the *pâte brisée?*

Anyone can enter the contest Madame Barthe originated. The pie can be sweet or savory and made with any ingredients, as long as garlic is one of them. Judges are chefs and food industry people, and they like originality and creative decoration as well as good taste. I like the pie decorated with a spray of carrots, made by a member of the carrot brotherhood. The winner, made by Lautrec's own Fernande Corbeil, is equally beautiful, judging by its photograph, but I don't see it until later; it's a zucchini and rice pie containing eight cloves of garlic, eggs, cheese, and a soupçon of tomato sauce, and the top is decorated with a large flower made of zucchini carved into petals and leaves and centered with a bulb of pink garlic.

THE WINNERS of the garlic art contest, judged early this morning, are on display in a room on the other side of Rue du

Mercadial, only a few steps away. But to get there we have to squeeze past a platoon of school majorettes twirling batons to a brass band and pick our way through a crowd that's gathered to watch the *manouille* contest. Tying a *manouille* for market is considered an art in France: the garlic stem is cut back to about 8 inches (20 centimeters), the roots are trimmed off, and the outer layers of skin are carefully removed until the glossy pink inner skin is exposed. Then the stems are wrapped and tied tightly together, stalk by stalk. It's the best way to package Lautrec's pink garlic because its stalks are rigid once the plants are cured. In the festival contest six growers take turns tying a giant *manouille* on long tables joined together under the loggia where we ate our bowls of soup only a couple of hours ago; the goal is to beat last year's record in a three-hour limit, but not by too much. This group is moving fast.

"If it gets too long it will be hard to beat the record the next year," says Pauline. "The aim is to progress regularly so it stays competitive."

The cook who can employ [garlic] successfully
will be found to possess the delicacy of perception,
the accuracy of judgment, and the dexterity of hand which
go to the formation of a great artist.
MRS. W.G. WATERS, author of *The Cook's Decameron:*
A Study in Taste (1901)

THE WINNING garlic sculpture is a 3-foot (1-meter) hot-air balloon made of overlapping translucent garlic skins floating over a garlic foliage landscape. Watching the balloon from below are garlic-bulb people wearing clogs carved from garlic cloves standing on a pathway made of chopped-garlic gravel edged with garlic-clove stones. Other entrants include an Eiffel Tower of garlic bulbs, and a life-size store mannequin dressed in a frothy gown of garlic skins. My favorite is the proud garlic rooster: he rises tall on realistic feet made of tiny garlic bulbils; his tail is a graceful sweep of garlic scapes; his comb and wattle shake their purple garlic skins. He stands regally displaying second prize, although in my mind he should have won first.

The rooster triggered thoughts of chicken in my subconscious, and I'm suddenly peckish. "Me too," says Chris, and we set out on a search for food. We look in vain for a food stall, because the booths in the marketplace are selling hats and jewelry, pottery, soaps, and rainbow-colored macaroons. A man is demonstrating a whiz of a garlic cutter, and I buy one. Eventually I see a man stirring a cauldron of a creamy white mixture. More soup? *Aligot*, says his sign.

"What is that?" I ask Pauline.

"*Aligot* is a specialty at festivals around here," she says. "It's mashed potatoes stirred and stirred with lots of fresh cheese till it gets really smooth. You buy a plastic plate of it and eat it with a spoon, or you get a container and take it home for dinner."

"May I have some?" I ask the man.

"*Non, non*, it's not ready yet," he says, stirring the mixture around and around, lifting it high into the air and then stirring more. When we return in half an hour it's smooth and elastic, ready for eating. Chris and I dip into a plateful.

"It needs garlic," I say.

"*Je regrette*," says the man. "I have none."

We remedy that easily enough—we return to the man demonstrating the garlic cutter, get a nice rounded spoonful of freshly chopped garlic, and stir it into our *aligot*. Now it's perfect, smooth and cheesy with a good hit of garlic, a concentrated purée of flavors. It holds us over until the *fabounade*, scheduled for seven-thirty in the *boulodrome* just outside the village walls, the grand finale of the day.

While we're changing for the event and having a glass of wine from Gaillac in our room, I eye the *manouille* I purchased at the shop yesterday, sitting on the mantel. Should I try to smuggle it home, or should I cut into a clove and sample it now, in case I get caught and thrown in jail and never get to taste it? I'm almost afraid to—what if I'm disappointed? But the garlic wins. I came here to find Ail Rose, and now that it's within my reach I have to see if it lives up to its billing.

I remove a clove, use my travel corkscrew to take off the skin, and bite down hard.

The garlic hits my wine-soaked tongue sharply but mellows out almost immediately. It's—different. Garlicky, naturally, but not strongly sulfurous. Sort of musky. The taste reaches a plateau and lingers beautifully.

I sigh with relief. It's good. But the flesh is creamy white, like that of every other garlic in the world. Was I really hoping it would be pink, like the skin? And what subgroup does Ail Rose belong to? To the French it's simply the best garlic in the world, and its subgroup is irrelevant. Just by looking at it I know it's not from the Artichoke subgroup, like Gilroy's 'California Early' with its many layers of bulging cloves and irregular shape. Ail Rose is compact and almost round, with each clove nearly identical in size and shape. It's perfect, as Madame Barthe says.

It's not until I get home and find a grower in the southern United States who lists 'Rose de Lautrec' on his website that I discover it's probably a Creole and originated in Spain. Perhaps that's where that mysterious medieval traveler came from with his precious garlic in his pocket, since Spain isn't far from this region of France. It's a fanciful story, but there may be some truth to it after all. Creoles are among the rarest of garlics and are sometimes difficult to find, and they're good to eat fresh because of their sweet, mellow flavor combined with heat. They're also known to last a long time, sometimes as long as the next year's harvest, in the right storage conditions.

As to whether I smuggled home the rest of the *manouille*, my lips are sealed.

A garlic caress is stimulating. A garlic excess soporific.
MAURICE EDMOND SAILLAND, aka Curnonsky

THE *FABOUNADE* is fabulous, even if we can't speak more than a few words to our fellow diners. I guess we look French enough because several people sit down beside us and try to strike up conversations. But they give up after *"Bonsoir"* or *"Joli soir"* and move off to find another location.

The thirteen hundred of us—moms and dads, grandmas and grandpas, and kids of all ages—sit on benches at long paper-covered tables. We sip local wine as a band from a nearby village travels around the tables playing universal favorites like "When the Saints Come Marching In." People clap and sing as we wait for the *confréries* to march in and dinner to begin.

In due time they arrive, moving slowly to their theme song. Then the *grande manouille* is carried in on planks held aloft by a dozen men and women. It's nearly 74 feet (22.5 meters), the longest in the festival's history and about 6½ inches (17 centimeters) longer than last year's. Now I realize why it can't get too much longer each year—the men and women of the garlic brotherhood wouldn't be able to carry it in.

Dinner, served by volunteers, is melon and ham followed by cassoulet topped with duck leg confit. It's a homey dish, the duck a bit overcooked and the white beans nicely soft and soupy. But as with the *aligot*, there isn't enough garlic. In fact, I don't think there's any. I have to remember we're in France, not Italy, and although the French like garlic, they never use it as liberally as Italians or even many North Americans, and sometimes not at all if they deem it unnecessary. Dessert is a square of lemon tart cut from a large bakery-made sheet. As Jacqueline Barthe would say, *comme ci, comme ça.*

As soon as the band strikes up after dinner, masses of people get up to dance. Women dance with women, children with children. And the men dance—they steer their partners expertly around the floor doing little box steps or waltzes, and they look happy about it.

But after a while we have nothing left to say to each other as well as no one else to talk to. It's time to leave. On the short walk back to our lodgings, I think about the evening. The menu wasn't the same, but the home-style meal reminded me of the turkey suppers held in Ontario villages and towns in the fall, the fried chicken fetes I've heard about in the southern states, or the summer lobster feasts and fish fries on the East Coast. But there was a difference: the French dinner had more joie de vivre. The French have their conservative, rule-following side, but then they totally abandon themselves to the enjoyment of food and wine and just being together in the moment. We could learn something from them.

The Canadian garlic festivals I've been to are informative, even educational, with lectures and demonstrations; unlike Gilroy and Lautrec, they offer many varieties of garlic to buy for planting or storing. The Canadian festivals are earnest and sincere and practical. Like Canadians? Gilroy's festival is pure Hollywood, but the organizers know how to run a big professional operation that's both slick and friendly, and the festival has made millions for local charitable organizations. The Fête de l'Ail Rose—well, it's French. It has innate style and class, plus a historical setting no place in North America can possibly match. Yet it's honest and down to earth; garlic is celebrated, but it stays suitably in the background. It's like a medieval fair without the bearbaiting and cockfighting.

I wonder what garlic festivals are like in Romania, where my little vegetable earned its reputation as a mighty vampire killer, or in Tajikistan, where it was first domesticated.

5

IN THE KITCHEN
WITH GARLIC

How to Chop, Preserve, and Cook with Garlic

Oh, holy to the nose
are the incense and sizzle that summon
folks from all parts of the house
to ask about dinner, sniffing...

DAVID YOUNG, *"Chopping Garlic"*

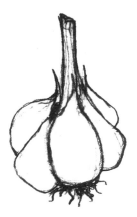

I noticed a long time ago that it wasn't until a clove was squashed in my garlic press that its unique fragrance suddenly bloomed and trumpets blared. I'm ashamed to say I never wondered why until a handful of years ago. Then I discovered that allicin, which gives garlic its unique taste and aroma—as well as most of its medicinal value—is created only when alliin (a sulfur compound known as S-allyl cysteine sulfoxide) and alliinase (an enzyme), which are contained in separate compartments inside the clove, come together. When a clove of garlic is cut or smashed, the two elements are released, producing allyl sulfenic acid, which immediately changes into allicin, chemically known as diallyl thiosulfate. It's a complicated chemical reaction, and it all happens in ten seconds.

More chemical reactions follow, releasing other compounds that contribute to garlic's taste as well as its therapeutic value. It's fascinating to realize that a mere smash of your knife can start a cascade of chemical interactions. This simple plant, which has been a kitchen staple for thousands of years, has become so important medicinally that scientists are studying it. We use garlic as often as onions and salt, but that doesn't mean we understand why it tastes the way it does or, more important, how the ways we prepare and cook it affect both its flavor and its benefits.

Raw garlic smashed and chopped finely or put through a press and used right away has, as experienced cooks know, the strongest taste. No, I'm wrong—a whole clove crushed by your very own teeth in your very own mouth has the strongest taste and the most therapeutic value, though not many people like their garlic that way.

The best way to get the ultimate flavor and greatest health benefits from garlic is to eat it raw or exposed to heat for as little time as possible. Raw garlic is a desirable taste in many sauces, spreads, and salads, such as aioli, chimichurri, pesto, tapenade, hummus, and tabbouleh, as well as cold soups like gazpacho and garlic-almond soup. Most of these dishes, you may notice, originated in warmer regions, such as the Mediterranean, South America, Spain, and the Middle East, where garlic was used as a preservative as well as a flavoring because of its antibacterial qualities—not, as many believe, because its strong taste disguised rotting food.

Some cooked dishes also benefit from a hit of raw garlic, like the easy pasta I sometimes make just for myself when Chris is off enjoying the company of his football buddies. It's a simple

• HOW MUCH GARLIC IS ENOUGH? •

The World Health Organization's guidelines recommend one clove a day to promote good health (cloves vary, so that's 0.07 to 0.18 ounces, or 2 to 5 grams); one clove seems to be the average daily consumption of garlic lovers. Garlic is an antioxidant, which reduces damage to the body caused by free radicals. One raw clove yields about 5 milligrams of allicin, the magical ingredient.

California author and garlic grower Chester Aaron swears by three cloves daily to keep him youthful and healthy, and to judge by his looks and work level, it works for him. He's eighty-eight and his twenty-seventh book was recently published. Ontario's Ted Maczka, the same age, still has plenty of vim and vigor; he eats three cloves a day.

Tests based on rats suggested that humans weighing 150 pounds (68 kilograms) could risk liver damage if they consume more than five cloves a day. The rats ate an equivalent amount for twenty-one days with no adverse effects, but there was significant liver deterioration after twenty-eight days.

Eating more than two cloves raw may irritate the stomach and esophagus, but this is hardly news. Eat raw garlic with food, in soup or hummus, or with bread.

Some people react badly to garlic, with severe breath and body odor, heartburn, and digestive upsets. These people may not be able to oxidize the sulfides in garlic into sulfoxides and may be wise to eat only cooked garlic.

concoction of leftover cooked linguine stirred with chicken stock, heavy cream, some grated lemon rind, and Parmesan cheese, with a chopped garlic clove tossed in just as the sauce thickens. Now that I know more about how garlic breaks down into that healthful allicin, I chop the garlic clove and let it sit for a few seconds, then remove the pan from the flame, let it cool a bit, and toss in the garlic. Even short contact with a bubbling hot sauce can kill the allicin. Along with a couple of grindings of black pepper, the garlic adds just the right kick to what could otherwise be an ordinary pasta dish. A soup or stew that's been cooked with a few spoonfuls of chopped garlic will have a more vivid flavor and therapeutic value if you drop in a little chopped raw garlic just before serving it or top each serving with a few bits. I like a little extra raw garlic on a nice big steak, too, even if it's been rubbed with garlic before cooking.

Garlic can taste almost any way you want it to,
depending on how you treat it.
LUCY WAVERMAN, food editor and cookbook author

Now that I buy and grow different cultivars and have a variety of garlic to choose from, I've learned to taste a bit of the one I'm going to use raw before tossing it in. Some varieties are hotter than others, and it is a good idea to make a few tasting notes as you experiment so you'll remember, say, that 'German Red' was just fine as a garnish on the goulash but that 'Susan Delafield' needs taming and is better roasted, unless you have a cast-iron tongue. In general, Creoles and Rocamboles—everyone's favorite garlic—have a sweeter, less hot flavor than Porcelains and

Silverskins. But there are exceptions among the cultivars; see "A Garlic Primer" for some guidelines.

RAW GARLIC is the perfect match for some foods, but other recipes, like the classic French chicken with forty cloves of garlic, require the mellow taste of whole cooked garlic cloves—and hang the therapeutic content. Garlic roasted as whole cloves to go with the Sunday roast contains no allicin or other sulfur compounds whatsoever. It's mellowed out, and many varieties that sting your mouth when raw lie down in lovely submission when cooked. This isn't a bad thing—there's nothing tastier than roasted garlic with the top cut off and olive oil poured over the exposed cloves. It's great smeared on a steak. Or blended into a wine sauce. Or mixed with olive oil and parsley and spread on toasted ciabatta. Roasted garlic may not have the health benefits of raw garlic, but who knows what other medicinal elements this amazing bulb produces when it's cooked?

Garlic that's crushed and chopped in even the most allicin-preserving way and then overbrowned in the sauté pan suffers the worst fate of all. Not only has the allicin been destroyed by the heat, the guts are fried out of the garlic taste, leaving it acrid and useless. Garlic should be gently sautéed till it's faintly tan and fragrant, and although that may not preserve the allicin, some of the other sulfur compounds will remain and the flavor will be developed, not ruined. Many recipes begin with onions being lightly browned in butter or oil, with garlic added as the onions properly color. I try to add the garlic at just the right moment so that both it and the onions develop their sweetness but aren't ruined by too much browning. It's a fine line.

Acids such as vinegar and lemon or lime juice also destroy allicin and much of garlic's taste. Remember this when you push a clove of garlic through your press directly into the vinegar in your vinaigrette. Push it into a bowl instead, or chop it on a board, and give it ten seconds to complete its magical transformation before adding it to an acid ingredient. Some of its compounds will be destroyed by the acid, but some will remain.

CHOPPING AND PREPPING

Chopping garlic is how I start dinner. It puts me in the mood for cooking and signals that the relaxed part of the day is nigh. Even the cats know it's time to meow for supper once they hear the knife and sniff that pungent smell. The smell of garlic makes everyone smile.

There's no special art to chopping garlic, but you have to do it a few times to get the hang of it. The first step, after freeing a clove from the bulb, is to get its tight little jacket off, the hardest part. You need strong fingers to squash the clove between thumb and forefinger to loosen the skin, but I've seen a few manly cooks do it. I used to cut the end off the clove and laboriously peel the skin off with my fingernails, a real drag with small cloves, but after seeing it in a movie a dozen years ago I adopted the knife smack common to today's TV chefs. This technique not only is more efficient but also makes you look like a pro: lay the clove on a board, place the flat of a chef's knife blade on top of it, and whack the knife with the heel of your hand. It's a bit messy, with skin scattering over the board like big dandruff flakes and the garlic lying in pieces, but it's the quickest way, and you can add variations to your whack. A light one provides a slightly flattened clove that might be just right for flavoring a Caesar dressing or some oil that needs just a faint garlic taste; a more murderous whack will squash the garlic like a fly and render it less in need of severe chopping.

If time isn't a problem, try soaking the cloves in a bowl of water for a couple of hours. The skin will pull off easily, leaving the cloves intact and perfect for sautéing or roasting (or for making chicken with forty cloves of garlic), and there will be no need for messy peeling at the table. The softneck varieties, which have tighter skins, require a good soak, after which you have to get your fingernail under one end of the clove to release the skin, but then it peels off nicely. Rocamboles and other hardneck types usually give up their coverings more easily.

There's another way to get the skin off: use one of those rubber squares sold to help unscrew tight lids. Fold the cloves in the rubber, press down, and roll back and forth. Voilà: skinned garlic. You can also buy a garlic roller-peeler some smart marketing person came up with to solve the problem. It's made of the same type of textured rubber and looks like a giant manicotti tube. It's well worth the few bucks it costs at most kitchen supply stores.

Once the clove is freed of its tight little jacket, start chopping. How to chop may seem elementary, my dear reader, but practice will make your technique look good and result in uniform pieces of garlic. Hold the handle of the knife with one hand and lay the palm of the other hand over the end of the blade, then rock the knife over the garlic. Move the handle end of the knife slightly as you cut to trace a quarter-circle shape on the board and cover all the garlic. The more you rock and move the knife back and forth, the finer the pieces will become. Scrape them up now and again and start over. It seems almost too obvious to mention, but finely minced garlic has more power and flavor than more coarsely chopped garlic.

"At Cordon Bleu they had us chop garlic with salt," says Lucy Waverman, food columnist and cookbook author. "It makes the garlic creamier, and it doesn't smell up the board as much. Once I chopped a lot of garlic in my food processor as a shortcut and then washed the bowl out and used it to make a dessert. Believe me, that was a big mistake."

With wooden boards, too, you need to wash everything well afterward to make sure the taste is gone. You might keep a special board for chopping garlic, or if you use the salt method, mash it in a mortar with a pestle or in a small bowl with the back of a spoon. A food processor chops garlic well if other ingredients are going to be added to the bowl, but it's useless for chopping a clove or two, because the garlic flies around and clings to the sides of the bowl and never reaches the texture you need.

TOOLS AND GADGETS

Does a kitchen exist without a garlic press? It was the first "exotic" culinary gadget I bought, years ago, and it made me feel as if I'd graduated from Cooking 101. Trouble was, it was cheap aluminum—and you know how bendable aluminum can be. Before long it looked like a pretzel. The next one was also aluminum, but industrial strength, and plain as a garbage can. It didn't even have a brand name, which most garlic presses seem to have these days.

That garlic press moved from house to house with me and lasted for at least thirty years. It did yeoman service until two springs ago, when Chris brought home a shiny new stainless steel one. It had no label, no identifying marks, a no-name press with no packaging. It was strong and beautiful, but by this time I'd graduated beyond the garlic press and was using a knife. And I felt pretty proud of myself for having advanced to this lofty plateau.

"I use my press only when I'm feeling incredibly lazy," says Lucy. "And then I have to wash the darn thing, and it's not easy getting those bits out. I control the texture of the garlic better when I chop it."

Aye to all those points. Cleaning the press was what made me perfect my cutting technique. When I discovered the different ways garlic tasted and looked when I used a knife, I left the garlic press behind.

But some garlic presses elicit superlatives from users— especially the Zyliss Susi, which was made in Switzerland way back when and now is manufactured in China. It comes in two models, one that hinges backward and has little protruding bits that push out the garlic residue, and a bigger model that holds more than one clove (try pressing down on that with an arthritic wrist!) and has a nonstick interior. Paul Pospisil of the *Garlic News* raves about the ratcheting garlic press sold by Lee Valley Tools, which is said to crush up to four cloves of skin-on garlic at a time with a light squeeze of the handle. The removable screen and swing-out plate reportedly make it easy to clean, too.

SOME COOKS use a rasp to grate garlic. It sounds like a good idea if you want finely grated cloves. I'd be careful of my fingers, though—garlic cloves aren't very big and they grate down

• GARLIC IN NAME ONLY •

Elephant garlic (*Allium ampeloprasum*) may look like a giant head of garlic, but it's a member of the leek family and grows to about twice its cousin's size. Many cooks like the convenience of its big cloves because less peeling is required for the same quantity, but this is a debatable advantage if you're after real garlic flavor; elephant garlic is milder and more oniony than true garlic. Some cooks prefer its taste, and others scorn it for being weak. Elephant garlic also produces less allicin than garlic. It does have one clear advantage over garlic, however: it has a longer shelf life at room temperature.

quickly, which could add a spot or two of blood to the dinner. A friend recently introduced me to a neat stainless steel rasp she'd bought at a kitchen store. It's a Microplane grater with a movable attachment that clamps over it with a knob on top and teeth underneath that hold the garlic (or ginger or nutmeg seed); you move it back and forth and the garlic is shredded finely. Garlic twisters, big at garlic fairs—where magicians demonstrate them and churn out bowls full of chopped garlic in seconds—are another option. I have two. Both are unnecessarily complicated, but one—the Nouveau Moulin à Ail, bought at the Fête de l'Ail Rose in Lautrec—turns out neat little squares of garlic without too much frustration. Chris likes it, but my knife is still faster.

But I do have a garlic-chopping friend that works better than my knife: the enigmatically named ulu. The Inuit made curved ulus in all sizes for removing seal skins and carving the meat, and I bet they never thought they'd see them used for chopping garlic. My ulu was given to me one Christmas by my daughter-in-law Chrissy, who loves garlic as much as I do. It's a simple 8-inch (20-centimeter) wood square (mine has inlaid strips of dark and light wood), with a round depression taking up most of the center; the half-moon blade is set in a wooden handle. The knife exactly fits the depression and makes mincemeat of the garlic in no time. It's the best garlic chopper I've ever used, and it also chops herbs beautifully. But remembering Lucy and her garlic-scented food processor, I scrub mine out frequently. I treat it to a good rub with vegetable oil about once a month, and I run a sharpening stone over the blade whenever it seems to need it.

Garlic keepers with (necessary) ventilation holes in the lid look neat on a shelf in the kitchen, but you don't really need them. Unglazed pots are better than glazed ones, but any container will do as long as the garlic is kept dry and ventilated. I store my garlic in an open bowl on a shelf above my spices. What looks more inviting than a garlic braid or rope hanging from the pot rack? Or a mesh vegetable bin filled with cloves? But don't expect to store a lot of garlic this way—in the warmth of your kitchen it will soon dry out. Keep only a month or two's worth of garlic on display.

Unglazed terra-cotta garlic roasters with domed lids are another nonessential garlic accessory, but they beat aluminum foil packages on a couple of counts. First, they roast the garlic bulbs or cloves at an even temperature and it's easier to scrape juices from their glazed bottoms than it is to struggle with a piece of crumpled super-hot foil. Second, they're much prettier. I prefer my roaster—which holds one large clove or two small ones.

This isn't the same as storing garlic in a cool place for as far into the winter as your varieties will keep. This is about being creative with drying and freezing or otherwise preserving your precious garlic crop, or the mountain of bulbs you bought at a garlic fair, so that you can keep it past its best-before date.

"But why would you bother?" says Lucy, and she has a point if you live in a city with greengrocers who care enough to buy good garlic from Mexico or Argentina once our domestic product is used up for the season. They might also buy from companies like Gilroy's Christopher Ranch that store their crop in climate-controlled warehouses to keep it fresh almost all year. But if you don't live in a more enlightened community, by the time January rolls around you'll have to settle for small supermarket garlic bulbs so old and badly stored they're either sprouting or turning to dust. That's when your very own preserved garlic is useful.

No one is indifferent to garlic.
People either love it or hate it, and most good cooks
seem to belong in the first group.
FAYE LEVY, food writer and cookbook author

WE HAVE a dry period from midwinter until the local new crop is ready, usually mid-August. Luckily I've been able to buy some pretty nice Purple Stripes from Argentina, where the seasons are nearly opposite to ours, so its garlic is ready when ours is done. But in the interests of research I've experimented with a few methods of preserving garlic, and I like freezing the best.

• WHEN GARLIC TURNS DEADLY •

Because garlic grows underground, it can contain spores of the soil-dwelling microorganism *Clostridium botulinum,* which causes deadly botulism poisoning, and garlic stored in oil offers it the perfect anaerobic home. Never store garlic in oil at room temperature. It's okay to prepare some garlic-infused oil for that night's vinaigrette, but throw out any unused portion. It may be fine the next day, but you may forget about it and keep it around for much longer.

The spores are resistant to heat, so cooking the garlic before putting it into the oil likely won't kill them. However, *C. botulinum* is sensitive to acid, so garlic cloves soaked in wine, vinegar, or citric acid for twenty-four hours can be stored in oil and kept in the refrigerator safely for about three months. Commercial garlic-and-oil products are prepared with acids under strict regulations to avoid the botulism threat.

Recently I thawed a few cloves that had spent a whole year in our deep freezer, which is colder than the freezer compartment of the fridge, and they were still strong and fresh. Like all frozen vegetables, they were a little translucent once thawed, but they retained a respectable amount of firm flesh.

There are several ways to freeze garlic, all of them dead easy. One is to immerse peeled whole or chopped cloves in water-filled ice cube trays and then put the frozen cubes in freezer bags. I put one whole clove or a teaspoon (5 mL) of chopped garlic in each tray section. I've thawed and roasted the whole cloves or dropped a whole cube into a soup I'm going to purée. The chopped garlic, thawed, works better for sautéing or in a stew or a regular soup where you don't want the presence of whole cloves. For sautéing, thaw the cubes of chopped garlic in a small dish and don't throw out the water—it's redolent of garlic and is a terrific addition to gravy or sauces.

Or you can purée garlic with oil and freeze it in small containers; use a ratio of about two parts oil to one of garlic. Because the oil doesn't completely freeze, you can spoon out what you need directly from the freezer. If you take the container out and it thaws and stays at room temperature for a length of time, don't use it (see the sidebar "When Garlic Turns Deadly").

The easiest way to freeze loose whole cloves is to leave the skin on and freeze them on a cookie sheet; then transfer them to containers. The next-easiest way is to peel them first. In my experience, both methods result in a softer, almost mushy texture compared with garlic frozen in water. But I suppose it hardly matters when you're going to be cooking them until they're soft.

Thawed garlic isn't so great as a substitute for raw garlic used as a garnish, though it works just fine in vinaigrette. So does a tablespoon (15 mL) of the garlic water.

Garlic is my desert island vegetable.

MICHAEL SMITH, cookbook author and Food Network host

DRYING GARLIC requires more attention and to my mind is less satisfactory than freezing, but if you have a lot of garlic and no deep freezer, it's the way to go. I've tried different methods—in

• WHEN GARLIC TURNS GREEN •

You need a background in chemistry to understand why garlic sometimes develops pretty blue or greenish spots. In his book, Eric Block says it's the result of a complex formation of pigments derived from several amino acids, not contact with the toxic salts of copper or cadmium, as some think, and it's perfectly safe to eat, though its flavor may be compromised.

In China this chemical process is used to produce green garlic, which is then pickled and served with dumplings at Chinese New Year celebrations.

the vegetable-and-fruit dehydrator that takes up space in my basement because I use it about every three years, in the microwave, and in the oven—and all kept the garlic well for several months. To start my experiment, I removed the skin from twenty cloves and sliced them about an eighth of an inch (0.4 centimeters) thick; that took nearly an hour and was the hardest part.

The dehydrator had no specific instructions for garlic, so I followed the general ones for potatoes, figuring garlic had about the same density and moisture content. I left the slices carefully laid out in the dehydrator for an hour at 97°F (36°C), then turned it up to 115°F (46°C) because I realized some summers are nearly that hot and it might take forever. After ten more hours they looked toasty and were brittle. After a month in a jar they'd softened a little but stayed strong, fragrant, and tasty until they were used by June of the following year.

IT'S DIFFICULT to get an ordinary electric oven down to just over 100°F (38°C), so I tried a couple of ways. First I heated the oven to 200°F (93°C)—the lowest mine will go—and left the slices in for seven minutes; then I turned off the oven and let the slices sit in it for a half-hour. I had toast-colored, very dry slices that looked brittle, but ten months later they still smelled strongly of garlic and reconstituted with good, if toasty, flavor. I let another batch sit an hour and fifteen minutes on a heated cast-iron pan in an oven preheated to 200°F (93°C) and then turned off before the garlic cloves went in, with the oven light left on to hold some heat. I liked them best at first—they were almost white and seemed properly dried, but although they retained their texture the flavor disappeared in about five months. A magazine article advised drying garlic cut in half at 140°F (60°C) for two hours and then lowering the temperature to 130°F (54°C) until the garlic pieces were totally dry and crisp. That seemed too much for the little guys, so I didn't try it; later I read that commercially processed garlic is dried at 122 to 140°F (50 to 60°C). Only above that temperature do flavors start to break down.

The microwave, with the garlic zapped for a minute at a time at high until the garlic was crisp, seemed the most successful drying method in the beginning. The slices were pearly white and full flavored, but they smelled like peanuts after about five months and had severely diminished flavor.

So you can see there's no hard-and-fast rule for drying garlic successfully. My most successful batch—if length of storage is a measure—was the first one (seven minutes with the heat on and half an hour in a turned-off oven). But all the garlic except the microwaved slices kept its goodness and flavor for as long as anyone might need.

The message is that you're on your own. Successful drying is a matter of experimentation, and results probably depend on the moisture content of the garlic and its variety, as well as how thin the slices are.

Garlic vinegar is another way to save the garlic from your garden for future use, but I don't think it's an effective option for preserving a lot of garlic—how much vinegar do you need in a year, anyway? Still, made with garlic from your own garden and put up in good-looking bottles with handmade labels, it's a great gift. Use wine vinegar, white or red, and drop in as many smashed or chopped cloves as you like. Add a sprig of rosemary or thyme and some peppercorns for appearance and extra taste, and you have an original dinner party gift.

GARLIC PRODUCTS

Garlic powder was the first garlic I cooked with because I knew nothing else, and it still has a place on my shelf. I think this shocked Lucy when I mentioned it. "I never use it," she said. "It's got a funny taste."

I agree it can't compare with fresh garlic, and sometimes it smells tinny to me in the package, but I find it useful. It's better than fresh chopped garlic for sprinkling over croutons made with day-old French bread, for example, or on the stale tortillas I cut into triangles and toast in the oven (my mother was a Depression-era cook and brought me up to be frugal) because it clings to the pieces and doesn't drop to the bottom of the bowl or storage bag, as pieces of chopped garlic do. Sometimes I add garlic powder to the gravy at the last minute when I have no time to chop some fresh.

Some beneficial attributes of fresh garlic are lost during the processing of garlic powder, but products vary and we have no way of knowing which are better. Some garlic powders bloom with that familiar garlic aroma when they meet a liquid, and I can only assume that some allicin is being produced. But because garlic is cut into pieces to help along the drying, some of the allicin has to be lost (the same is true of your home-dried garlic; the allicin retained in frozen garlic is a big question mark). And although garlic powder has a definite garlic taste—most of it is about two and a half times as potent as fresh garlic—it doesn't have the nuanced flavor of fresh garlic, perhaps because processing produces some sulfur compounds that don't exist in fresh garlic.

Peeled garlic cloves that come in a jar or plastic bag are a recent innovation that look like the best invention since the garlic press, but I'm from Missouri. Can life really be this easy? How can they possibly stay fresh and tasty for however long it takes them to get from there to here without going moldy? What are they steeped in anyway? I bought some to find out. I chopped a clove on my ulu, and it had no smell or taste—well, okay, it had a *little* smell and taste. Then I chopped a fresh clove of garlic, and the difference came home. The processed cloves have a certain appeal, no doubt, but they've been so blanched and acidified to stay fresh and looking good that they're nearly useless. Their flavor is compromised, as well as their therapeutic benefits.

Let's face it: all methods of processing garlic so that it fits into jars or packages are going to deplete some of its goodness. Garlic powder or dehydrated garlic (used mainly in health supplements and convenience foods) or peeled or chopped garlic in jars is convenient, but it isn't the same as fresh garlic. It doesn't taste the same and doesn't have the same nutritional or therapeutic value, and we shouldn't kid ourselves that it does. But if it's what you need at the time, use it.

TRENDY GARLIC

Garlic is a hot commodity. Sometimes I fear it's in danger of becoming so trendy it will turn into tomorrow's oat bran. I believe the basic garlic bulb will endure for another ten thousand years or more because of its value as a flavoring and its health benefits; it's the fancy garlic parts that may be passing fancies.

Take garlic scapes, the flower stalks of hardneck varieties of garlic, which are usually removed sometime in June, before their lovely curling shape straightens. A few years ago no one had heard of scapes, but now they're considered a rare delicacy and sell for high prices—in the summer of 2011 they were priced at a quarter each or five for a dollar at the Friday farmers' market near my house. Can you imagine green beans selling individually? Five summers ago that same farmer would have thrown those scapes onto the compost heap. But they've caught the fancy of food editors everywhere, and every spring newspapers and magazines run the latest methods for cooking them, and websites and blogs rave about the virtues and plate appeal of this latest trendy vegetable. Restaurants love scapes—they're different, they look good, and they signal that this establishment is on top of the food trends.

Perhaps I'm being churlish, but I think there's a whiff of the emperor's new clothes in the scape's status as a delicacy. It

• GOT GARLIC BREATH? •

The strong odor caused by garlic starts in the mouth, extends to the gut, and finally is exuded by the lungs and through sweat, and it's probably going to last thirty hours no matter how often you use mouthwash. The odor is caused by various sulfides produced when garlic is digested.

The classic remedy is to chew parsley, but eating any of several raw fruits and vegetables, such as kiwi, basil, eggplant, mushrooms, and spinach, helps neutralize the effect. Cooked rice, cow's milk, or eggs can also help. But when it comes down to it, your friends will probably have to wait it out until the garlic leaves your body.

You could try a sauna, though—a good sweat might speed up the process.

makes an interesting, mildly garlicky dip when chopped finely and combined with sour cream or thick Greek yogurt, and it's okay but a bit tough chopped into lengths and simmered in olive oil. But scapes don't taste even a bit like asparagus to me, despite all the blogs I've read. I admit that they taste better—and don't seem as tough—quickly parboiled and then bathed in olive oil and grilled on the barbecue, which adds flavor of its own. But I don't think garlic-scape pesto compares with the real thing, the one made with basil and lots of garlic and pine nuts, though Lucy says I should add grated lemon rind and some bread crumbs to enhance the flavor and texture. I'll try that next year.

Like many cooks, I didn't know what to do with the pointy ends of the scapes—the immature flower bud ends. Were they edible? Should I cut them off? But they are the most attractive part of the scape, so I left them on. Actually, they had more taste than the rest of the stalk, but they were tougher, and the rough, sort of crumbly texture wasn't exactly pleasant. The next time I cut them off, chopped them up finely, and sprinkled them over the sautéed stems. That was better.

I WILL admit that the popularity of scapes has probably made life better for small growers. It must be a chore to have to cut each one off to allow the bulbs to reach their full size, and selling them to eager customers must be a way to offset some of the labor costs. Typically, the scapes are cut after they've coiled downward and have that nice curl customers like but before they straighten and point upward. Holding off until this precise time is thought to allow the bulbs to last longer in storage. But if they were cut before they curled at all, not long after they'd emerged from the underground stem, they would be more tender. Home growers could easily cut scapes at this desirable earlier point because it's probably not as important for their garlic to have long storage capability. I read somewhere that in Italy it's common practice among commercial growers to grow some garlic just for its scapes. This could be the next step here, too.

A couple of kinds of green garlic are also becoming popular. Garlic scallions are, like onion scallions, young plants grown for their tender leaves and tiny bulbs, which have a delicate, slightly garlicky taste. They're a treat, and they can be grown in a pot on your windowsill for winter or in the garden for fall, planted as soon as you harvest your crop in July. Very small cloves are ideal for this purpose, as are large bulbils from a mature scape, planted an inch (2.5 centimeters) or less apart. Use a good potting soil in your indoor pot, and add some well-rotted compost to the outdoor patch. Like scapes, garlic scallions can be grilled or pan-fried, methods that bring out their sweetness, and they're good in stir-fries or raw in salads. The tops that grow from rounds— the garlic plants that may have gone wild in your garden and haven't yet developed multicloved bulbs—are also good eaten as garlic scallions.

Garlic scallions are often called green garlic, but true green garlic is actually a little different. It's more mature than the scallion but not quite grown up yet. It's not as intensely flavorful as mature garlic and doesn't have the scallion's tender and milder attributes, and the bulb may contain a few pristine cloves with the many layers of skin still undeveloped. It's sold whole, with the bulb and the green tops intact, mainly in farmers' markets, though some larger greengrocers in the United States sell them.

Garlic greens, as opposed to green garlic, are more mature plants and are yet another way to eat garlic. In tropical countries, garlic is frequently grown just for its tops, since garlic doesn't form bulbs in hot climates. Garlic greens aren't often seen in North America, however, if at all. As an experiment you could try growing some to add to stews as you would cabbage or kale. I bet they'd make a fine soup, too. Plant small cloves for the smallest and tenderest greens and harvest before the leaves become tough—but be warned they're not going to be as tender as garlic scallions. Once they reach a foot (30 centimeters), it's time to get out the scissors.

The reverse snob in me was prepared to heartily dislike fermented black garlic, the latest and hottest trend. It appeared out of nowhere in a San Francisco gourmet food shop in 2008; then it was used on *Top Chef: New York* and *Iron Chef America*. In 2008 it was listed in the American trade publication *Nation's Restaurant News* by chef Matthias Merges of Charlie Trotter's restaurant in Chicago as one of his five food finds of the year. A few months later the *Washington Post* ran an article about it, followed by the Toronto *Globe and Mail*. Oh, there was more. The best shops—and only the best ones—started stocking it. I looked for it and couldn't find it. I realized I shopped at the wrong stores and decided I wouldn't bother.

Yes, I dug my heels in. But when I finally found it, selling at two bulbs for five dollars, took it home and spread two cloves on crusty rolls under tomato slices, roasted red peppers, fresh mozzarella and prosciutto, I ate my words as well as the sandwich. It was sweet, creamy, fruity, smoky.

"Mmmm, did you put some kind of balsamic sauce on this?" asked Chris. "I like it."

A few people tried to tell me that fermenting garlic was an ancient method of preserving it and that eating fermented garlic guarantees a long life. I checked it out and it isn't true, or at least it's unprovable. Fermented black garlic was invented by Scott Kim in South Korea in 2004 as a health product. I'd love to know how he came up with the idea. He used a forty-day heat-curing process that leaves the bulbs slightly shrunken but with still-white skins. The cloves inside are black, soft, and chewy. Kim says his garlic contains twice as many antioxidants as fresh garlic, as well as S-allyl cysteine, a factor reported to play a role in preventing some types of cancer.

Now that I've tried black garlic on sandwiches as well as pasta—mashed into a sauce made with cream and mushrooms—I'm wondering how to use it in other ways. The website (see "Sources") offers several recipes, including an Asian-style salad with noodles and vegetables and a dish of scallops and chorizo, that sound good.

Black garlic and all the other variations I mention here prove my belief that garlic is being reborn. It's appearing in grocery stores and on cooking shows in many different guises. It's gaining respect as more than a folk remedy or a homeopathic cure but as a plant with serious therapeutic value. Yet it remains that odorous, delicious, spellbinding, magical potion I discovered in an Italian restaurant long ago. After all is said and done, the best thing to do with garlic is to eat it, however it is served.

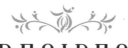

RECIPES

Warm-Weather Watermelon Crabmeat-Kissed South Seas Soup

Margee Berry of Trout Lake, Washington, won first prize at the 2010 Gilroy Garlic Festival with this delicious cold soup. Its fresh, fruity sweetness is beautifully balanced with a hit of garlic, the tang of lemongrass and lime juice, and a bit of heat provided by fresh ginger and chilies.

I wasn't able to get blood oranges when I made this in summer, so I used regular oranges, squeezed fresh. The taste is just a touch sweeter. *Serves 6*

5 cups	cubed seedless watermelon
1 tbsp	mild olive oil
1/4 cup	chopped shallots
2 tsp	peeled and minced ginger
2 tsp	trimmed and minced fresh lemongrass *(see Note)*
1 tsp	minced Thai chili or other hot chili, such as serrano
1 tbsp	minced garlic
1 cup	freshly squeezed blood orange juice
2 tsp	rice vinegar
1 tsp	fish sauce
1/2 tsp	sea salt

CRABMEAT TOPPING

2 cups	cooked lump crabmeat
1/4 cup	finely chopped green onion
3 tbsp	chopped cilantro
2 tbsp	chopped fresh mint
2 tsp	fresh lime juice
4 tbsp	grated radish

In a blender, purée the watermelon, then transfer to a large bowl. Set aside.

Heat oil in a large saucepan over medium-high heat and add the shallots, ginger, lemongrass, and chili; sauté 5 minutes. Add garlic and sauté 1 minute more. Transfer to blender along with orange juice, vinegar, fish sauce, and salt; purée until smooth. Stir into watermelon purée, then strain mixture and press it through a fine sieve into another bowl. Discard solids. Chill soup for at least an hour to blend flavors.

CRABMEAT TOPPING: In a medium bowl, toss together drained (if canned) crabmeat, green onion, cilantro, mint, and lime juice.

TO SERVE: Ladle soup into 6 bowls. Mound about 1/3 cup of crabmeat mixture in center of soup and garnish top of crabmeat with grated radish. Serve at room temperature or slightly chilled.

NOTE: Trim root end off lemongrass and remove 2 outer leaves. Finely mince with a Microplane zester or a knife. Ginger and garlic can also be minced on the Microplane.

Sopa de Ajo Blanco

Chris and I ate this soup in almost every restaurant we visited while we were in Spain, and each was a little different. It's bracing, smooth, and spicy but with a sweet edge provided by the grapes, and it's especially appealing on a hot day. This is my version, and I change the amount of garlic almost every time I make it—the number of cloves depends on how big they are and whether you're in the mood for mellow or intense. *Serves 6*

4 slices	white bread without crusts *(any kind)*
3/4 cup	blanched ground almonds
5 or 6 cloves	garlic, chopped
1/4 cup	extra-virgin olive oil
2 tbsp	sherry vinegar
2 cups	water
2 cups	chicken stock
	salt to taste
	about 1/2 lb seedless green or red grapes

Put bread in a bowl and cover with water. Allow to sit a couple of minutes, then drain and squeeze out as much water as you can. Crumble bread and put in food processor with almonds, garlic, oil, vinegar, and water. Process until smooth. Transfer to a bowl and blend in chicken stock. Taste and add salt as needed. Chill well. To serve, put some grapes in the bottom of each bowl and pour soup over.

Cold-Coming-On Soup

"This is just too incredibly simple," says my friend Pat. "But it's a great cold remedy," says her husband, Ian. The general rule is six cloves of garlic for each cup of stock, plus one for the pot. *Serves 2*

13 cloves	garlic, peeled
2 cups	chicken stock *(or beef or vegetable, but the legendary chicken fights colds)*
2 thick slices	crusty bread
	grated Gruyère or cheddar cheese

Simmer garlic in stock 15 to 20 minutes, or until tender. Blend with immersion blender.

Put bread into bowls and sprinkle it with the cheese. Pour the soup over, wrap yourself in a blanket, hold the bowl close to your mouth so that you smell the vapors, and spoon it in.

Potage de l'Ail Rose

How can a soup so easy taste so delicious? This soup draws crowds at Lautrec's Fête de l'Ail Rose the first Friday of every August, where 250 gallons is made to feed the throng. The pink garlic, of course, contributes to the flavor, but it's not widely available in North America; use a mild Rocambole or other garlic instead. *Serves 4*

2 quarts	water
10 cloves	garlic
5 ounces	vermicelli
1	egg, separated
1 tsp	mustard, preferably Dijon
	olive oil *(approximately 1 cup)*
	salt and pepper to taste

In a large saucepan bring the water to a boil. Crush the garlic and chop the cloves finely or put them through a garlic press. Add to the water all at once. Stir the egg white to a froth and add to water, whisking all the time. Simmer 3 minutes. Break vermicelli into short pieces, add to broth, and simmer another 3 minutes.

To make a mayonnaise, use a food processor, blender, or whisk to beat egg yolk with mustard. Add oil in a slow stream until mixture emulsifies and becomes creamy; you'll use close to a cup.

Slowly add a ladleful of warm stock to mayonnaise, then delicately fold mayonnaise into the soup. Season to taste.

Lentil, Bacon, and Tomato Stew with Forty Cloves of Garlic

"Garlic lovers, this dish is for you," says Michael Smith, an award-winning cookbook author, Food Network host, and Prince Edward Island's official food ambassador. "It includes garlic two different ways with two different flavors: pungent and mellow. The lentil stew is earthy, simmered with bacon and roasted garlic; then it's finished with a sizzling last-second dose of freshly sautéed garlic." Serve with roasted Yukon Gold potatoes. *Serves 6*

40 cloves	peeled garlic, 30 cut in half, 10 minced
1/4 cup	olive oil
8 slices	bacon, sliced crosswise into small strips
1	large onion, chopped finely
1	carrot, diced small
1 cup	green or Puy lentils
4 cups	chicken broth or water
one 28-ounce can	diced tomatoes
1 tsp	dried thyme
2 tsp	vinegar, any kind
	a sprinkle or two of salt and lots of freshly ground pepper

Preheat oven to 350°F. In a small ovenproof dish, toss the garlic cloves with 2 tbsp of the oil. Roast the cloves, stirring once, until they're golden brown, about 30 minutes. Reserve.

Meanwhile make the stew. Cook bacon until crisp in a large pot over medium-high heat. Transfer to a few folded paper towels to drain. Pour off and discard all but 1 to 2 tbsp of the bacon fat. Add onion and carrot to the pot and sauté, stirring frequently, until they're tender, about 5 minutes. Add lentils, broth, tomatoes, and thyme and bring to a boil. Reduce heat and simmer until the lentils are tender, about 40 minutes. When the roasted garlic cloves are done, stir them in.

Just before serving, stir in the bacon and vinegar. Season to taste with salt and pepper. Splash the remaining oil into a sauté pan over medium-high heat. Add the minced garlic and sauté, stirring occasionally until it begins to brown, 3 or 4 minutes. Pour the sizzling garlic oil with the garlic bits over the surface of the soup.

MICHAEL'S HINT: Roast the garlic cloves slowly to remove their pungency and bring out a deep aromatic flavor. The splash of vinegar adds brightness and enhances the flavors without announcing its sour presence. *(From* Chef Michael Smith's Kitchen, *Penguin, 2011; used with permisssion.)*

Perplexed Portobello Steak with Mushroom Purée and Mushroom Crudo

"The portobellos should almost caramelize in the pan juices so they taste rich, like steak," said Ryan Scott, executive chef at Ryan Scott 2 Go in San Francisco, who won the 2010 Gilroy Garlic Festival's Celebrity Showdown with this vegetarian dish. "I call it perplexed because they don't know whether they're meat or mushrooms." There's just enough garlic in the purée and crudo to enhance the earthy taste.   *Serves 2*

MUSHROOM PURÉE

1 tbsp	extra-virgin olive oil
1 tbsp	unsalted butter
2	shallots, minced
1/2 pound	cremini mushrooms, finely diced
1/2 pound	fresh shiitake mushrooms, trimmed and finely diced
1 tsp	minced fresh thyme
1/2 cup	vegetable stock
1 tbsp	sherry vinegar
	salt and freshly ground pepper to taste

Heat a sauté pan over medium-high heat and add oil and butter. Sauté the shallots until translucent, about 1 minute. Add the mushrooms and thyme and cook over moderate heat until the mushroom liquid evaporates, about 10 minutes. Add stock and vinegar, bring to a boil, and simmer briskly until thick, 7 to 10 minutes. Season to taste. Carefully transfer mixture to a blender and purée until smooth but still thick. Refrigerate until ready to use.

MUSHROOM CRUDO

1/2 cup	thinly sliced mushrooms
1/4 cup	finely diced red onion
1 tsp	finely chopped garlic
2 tbsp	finely chopped green garlic
1 tbsp	finely chopped parsley
1 tsp	sherry vinegar
3 tbsp	extra-virgin olive oil
	salt and freshly ground pepper to taste

In a bowl combine mushrooms, onion, both kinds of garlic, parsley, and vinegar. Stream in olive oil, stirring well. Season to taste.

PORTOBELLO STEAKS

2	whole portobello mushrooms
1 cup	vegetable broth
½	small onion, diced
1 clove	garlic, minced
3 tbsp	balsamic vinegar
1 tbsp	white wine
1 tsp	chopped thyme
½ tsp	chopped rosemary
1 tbsp	extra-virgin olive oil

Remove stems from mushrooms (and discard or reserve for another use) and set caps aside. Pour a thin layer of the vegetable broth into a large frying pan, add onion and garlic, and cook 2 minutes over high heat. Add remaining ingredients, except mushroom caps, and turn heat to medium. Add mushrooms, cover, and cook 5 minutes. Gently flip mushrooms over and cook another 5 minutes, adding broth as needed to prevent sticking. Place mushrooms on a large plate and spoon pan juices on top.

TO ASSEMBLE: Place a swirl of Mushroom Purée on each of 2 plates. Lay a Portobello Steak on each plate and top with Mushroom Crudo.

Salsa Verde

"I use this salsa with fish, strewn over a tomato salad, or with grilled chicken," says Lucy Waverman. "Occasionally I dot it over a pizza, too." *Makes about 1 cup*

1/3 cup	coarsely chopped Italian parsley
2 tbsp	capers
1 clove	garlic
3	anchovy fillets
2 tbsp	fresh bread crumbs
1 tbsp	lemon juice
1/2 cup	olive oil
	salt and freshly ground pepper to taste

Place parsley, capers, garlic, anchovy fillets, and bread crumbs in food processor. Process until finely chopped. Add lemon juice and olive oil and process until just combined. Add salt and pepper to taste.

Four Thieves Vinegar

During the seventeenth century doctors and priests carried garlic to protect them from plague, which was spread by fleas. Four thieves released from prison to collect the dead went further: they wore face masks soaked in garlic, vinegar, and herbs, and they didn't catch the disease and die, as expected. This recipe is an adaptation, without the wormwood and rue of the original.
Makes 4 cups

1/2	cinnamon stick
1	whole nutmeg
4 cloves	garlic, peeled
4	whole cloves, crushed
1 sprig each	rosemary, sage, mint, and lavender
4 cups	red wine vinegar

Put all ingredients in a large jar and stand in a sunny window for a month. Strain and seal. Good in vinaigrettes, soups, or stews; to deglaze a pan after sautéing beef or chicken; or to chase away the bugs that cause plague.

Les Blank's Lunch

"I favor the whole-wheat walnut bread I buy at Acme Bread in Berkeley," says the documentary filmmaker, who released the exuberant *Garlic Is as Good as Ten Mothers* in 1980. "But any hearty full-grain bread will do." You could put a slice on top and make this a full sandwich, but it looks more delicious when it's left open face. *Serves 1*

1	organically grown 'Early Girl' tomato, thickly sliced
1/2	avocado, sliced
1 thick slice	hearty, healthy bread
1 tsp	finely chopped garlic
	extra-virgin olive oil

Lay the slices of tomato and avocado on the bread and sprinkle the garlic over. Drizzle with as much or as little olive oil as you like.

Whole-Hog Potatoes

John Melone, son of Rudy Melone, one of the founders of the Gilroy Garlic Festival, says he became a surgeon so that he'd be good enough with a knife to cook at the festival. He made these garlicky potatoes on stage and used them as a bed for a side of smoked salmon. "I used unpeeled red potatoes and mashed them with the skins on for the color," he says. "But I also like to use peeled Yukon Golds—they're waxy and give a thicker, buttery texture—or russets, which are crumbly and flakier." *Serves 8*

6 to 8	medium potatoes
4 cloves	garlic, peeled
1 stick (½ cup)	unsalted butter
½ cup	grated cheddar or
	Monterey Jack cheese
¼ to ½ cup	heavy cream
	chopped green garlic, if you have it

Boil potatoes and garlic together. Drain and put back on warm element to dry off. Add butter and mash well. Add cheese while potatoes are still hot. Stir in cream until consistency is fluffy. Fold in chopped green garlic.

Jacqueline Barthe's Creamy Garlic Pie

Mme Barthe's favorite family supper inspired the pie competition at the Fête de l'Ail Rose in Lautrec, France. "We all adore this pie," says her granddaughter, Pauline Danigo. "We'd eat it any time, all day, not just for supper." *Serves 6 or 8*

	pâte brisée for 1-crust pie
2 ounces	butter, cold and cubed
2 ounces	grated Parmesan cheese
10 cloves	garlic, peeled and sliced thinly
2 ½ ounces	pine nuts
4	eggs
¾ cup plus 2 tbsp	crème fraîche

Roll out pâte brisée and fit into tarte pan with removable bottom. Trim edge flush with top of scalloped edge of pan. With fingers or fork, mix butter and cheese until crumbly. Sprinkle evenly over pastry. Top with garlic slices and pine nuts. Beat eggs and stir in crème fraîche. Pour evenly over base. Bake in 350°F oven about 40 minutes. "My grandmother says to be sure to keep checking as it cooks," says Pauline. "The filling is thin and could easily burn."

Roasted Garlic, Blueberry, and Pear Cobbler with Garlic-Pecan Brickle Cream

Yes, garlic in dessert! This yummy one from Penny Malcolm of Americus, Georgia, didn't place in the 2010 Gilroy Garlic Festival Great Garlic Cook-Off, but it sure tastes like a winner. The roasted garlic gives it a warm and savory undertone you don't expect to encounter in a sweet dish. *Serves 6*

1/2 cup	unsalted butter
two 15-ounce cans	sliced pears in natural juice
2 cups	fresh or frozen blueberries
2 cups	sugar
1/2 cup	water
6 cloves	roasted garlic, puréed
2 cups	self-rising flour
3 cups	buttermilk
1 tsp	pumpkin-pie spice
1 tsp	vanilla

GARLIC-PECAN BRICKLE CREAM

½ cup	sugar
¼ cup	light corn syrup
¼ cup	water
½ cup	chopped pecans
1 tbsp	unsalted butter
¼ tsp	vanilla extract
¼ tsp	baking soda
	pinch of salt
1 clove	roasted garlic, puréed
1 ½ cups	whipping cream
¼ cup	sugar

Preheat oven to 450°F. Put butter in a 13 × 9 × 2-inch baking dish and put dish in oven to melt butter and get it hot. While butter is heating, put pears with their juice, blueberries, 1 cup of the sugar, and the 1/2 cup water in a large microwave-safe bowl and microwave on high 3 to 4 minutes until the sugar has dissolved and the liquid is hot. Add roasted garlic and stir well. In another large mixing bowl, whisk together the flour, buttermilk, pumpkin-pie spice, vanilla, and remaining cup of sugar.

Remove the baking dish from the oven. The butter should be sizzling but not browned. Pour the batter evenly over the melted butter without stirring. Spoon the fruit and juices over the batter without stirring. Bake 15 minutes, then lower oven temperature to 350°F. Bake 45 minutes longer, or until the crust has risen to the top and turned golden brown.

Let cobbler cool slightly before serving to allow the juices to thicken.

GARLIC-PECAN BRICKLE CREAM: While cobbler is cooking, prepare the brickle. Cook ½ cup sugar, corn syrup, and 1/4 cup water in a small heavy-bottomed saucepan over medium heat 3 to 4 minutes, until sugar has dissolved. If sugar adheres to the side of the pan, brush it down with a pastry brush dipped in a little water. Add pecans and cook, stirring often, to 300°F on a candy thermometer. Remove pan from heat and add remaining ingredients except for the whipping cream and ¼ cup sugar; quickly pour mixture onto a piece of oiled parchment paper and allow it to cool completely. When it's cool, chop into small pieces.

Whip the cream until frothy. Add sugar and whip until it forms stiff peaks. Fold in brickle, reserving a few pieces for garnish.

Serve cobbler warm, topped with the whipped cream mixture and garnished with a few pieces of brickle.

A GARLIC PRIMER

What to Plant and How It Tastes

G*arlic has been* around for so long and traveled the world so widely that it's almost impossible to classify its numerous descendants, especially now that it's become a vegetable of interest and growers are developing new cultivars. Nevertheless, scientists, taxonomists, and breeders are trying to pin down its lineage. Over the past twenty-five years research into the genetics of garlic has been intense and classifications have changed more than once.

Although genetics may not matter much to the home gardener, it can make interesting reading (see "Sources" for a couple of books on the subject) and will eventually have an impact on the garlic we grow and eat. The number of cultivars has been increasing every year since 1989, when Russia allowed the United States Department of Agriculture into the country to gather samples, which have subsequently entered the North American market. It's enough to say there's a lot more garlic out there than you know about. If you want variety in your repertoire, go to garlic fairs or consult the websites of growers who sell garlic for seeding and eating.

Today garlic is divided into two main types: hardneck (*Allium sativum* var. *ophioscorodon*), which grows a scape or flower stalk, and softneck (*A. sativum* var. *sativum*), which doesn't. Hardneck garlic includes eight subgroups, and softneck garlic includes two subgroups (see below). These ten subgroups include dozens of cultivars; these are the named varieties we see when we buy from growers.

Just to complicate things, three of the hardneck subgroups (Asiatic, Turban, and Creole) don't always grow a scape, and if they do it will be less woody than the scapes of most hardneck varieties; for this reason they are sometimes referred to as weakly bolting hardnecks. ("Bolting" is a term generally used to describe the premature growth of a flower stem among cool-weather plants, such as spinach and lettuce, which can run to seed early in hot weather.) Generally speaking, the softneck and weakly bolting hardneck cultivars do better in the milder climates of Canada and the United States, and true hardnecks are recommended for areas with cold winters. But be bold and experiment: garlic is a survivor and if given a chance can adapt to growing conditions anywhere except the Arctic and the deep tropics.

Here's an arbitrary list of a few favorite cultivars, arranged under main type and subgroup. There are plenty more around. A couple of caveats: the tasting notes are subjective, gleaned from my notes and the tasting notes of others. The conditions under which garlic grows affect its taste as well as the color of the skins. Depending where you live, the cultivars mentioned here might not be available at your local fair or grower, but others just as good will be.

It's always better to start with proven cultivars sold by growers in your area and then to branch out and try more "exotic" varieties from other parts of the country, available through catalogs. See "Sources" for a sampling of growers who sell by mail and for a listing of a few garlic festivals and fairs.

Hardneck

ROCAMBOLE

Every cook's favorite. Excellent raw—less sulfurous, mellower, and sweeter than many other garlics. Rocamboles need cold winters to grow well and may not grow at all where winters are mild. Easy to peel, but the looser skins mean they don't store long.

'Brown Saxon':
    Plump, brownish cloves; strong rich flavor.
'German Red':
    Light tan cloves with a bit of purple at the base. Hot raw; retains strong garlic taste when cooked.
'Killarney Red':
    Might be a child of 'German Red' or 'Spanish Roja'; large cloves; rich, full flavor.
'Puslinch' (also called 'Ontario Giant'):
    Robust, lively flavor.

'Russian Red':
>   Deep, sweet, full flavor. Brought to Canada by
>   Doukhobors in late 1800s.

'Spanish Roja':
>   Large bulbs, rich, full, spicy flavor, a big favorite;
>   mellow when cooked; needs cold winters.

PURPLE STRIPE

Named for the striped skin, this subgroup is genetically closest to the original garlic. Some varieties still produce seed. Longer storing than Rocamboles, they also need cold winters to produce well and will grow in poor soil. Plump cloves.

'Chesnok Red' *(also called 'Shvelisi')*:
>   From the Republic of Georgia. Rich yet sweet;
>   excellent roasted or sautéed.

'Persian Star' *(also called 'Samarkand')*:
>   Brought to North America from a bazaar in 1989.
>   Rich flavor, medium bite, sweet and mellow when
>   roasted.

GLAZED PURPLE STRIPE

Bulbs are squat, shiny, and purplish, with faint stripes and large cloves, but they're no relation—except in the larger sense of being garlic—to Purple Stripes. In fact, DNA studies show that the Asiatics are closer to Glazed Purple Stripes than are the Purple Stripes. (I told you the study of garlic was complicated.)

'Purple Glazer':
>   Collected in the Republic of Georgia.
>   Sweet, hot, and rich.

'Red Rezan':
> From Russia, southeast of Moscow. Good garlic
> flavor on the mild side.

'Vekak':
> A more intensely flavored cultivar; reportedly
> especially rich when sautéed to a golden color.

MARBLED PURPLE STRIPE

Most experts agree this is not a subgroup of Glazed Purple Stripe but another horticultural subgroup, and the name describes its dappled, striped skin. Plants are vigorous and tall with strong, dramatically curling scapes. They do well in cold climates but have been known to adapt to warmer areas, such as Texas, where one grower reported a good crop.

'Bogatyr':
> Large, long-storing bulbs; very hot with a strong
> garlic taste when raw, especially when grown in
> southern climates, where it usually performs well.
> Taste remains fairly strong when cooked.

'Metechi':
> Late maturing, long storing; produces well in
> regions with mild winters as well as colder ones;
> hot and strong.

PORCELAIN

These are statuesque plants with thick stems—more correctly called pseudostems. Bulbs are large and white, with a few large cloves. Porcelain garlic produces more allicin and thus a stronger taste than other varieties. Very cold hardy but adaptable to milder climates. Good soil is important, as is sufficient water, even just before harvest time.

'Dan's Russian':
A variety developed on Salt Spring Island in British Columbia. Strong yet mellow flavor enhanced by cooking.

'Fish Lake #3':
A robust cultivar developed by Ontario's Ted Maczka, with a strong, lasting garlic flavor.

'Georgian Crystal':
Another from the Republic of Georgia. Less biting than some Porcelains.

'Georgian Fire':
A hot one, also from Georgia. Flavor lingers.

'Majestic':
Developed in eastern Ontario. A lovely big bulb with good-sized cloves and a full garlicky taste.

'Music':
A strong, dependable grower brought from Italy and now seen frequently at fairs in parts of Canada. Its big cloves are hot and pungent when raw, mellow when baked, although texture isn't as creamy as that of some other cultivars.

'Romanian Red':
Among the first Porcelains to arrive in North America more than a century ago. High allicin yield; pungent and hot raw with a more complex flavor when roasted.

'Rosewood':
> From Poland. Strong, lingering flavor.

'Susan Delafield':
> Hot; grows well in British Columbia and isn't averse to damp conditions.

ASIATIC

Previously considered related to the Artichoke subgroup of soft-necks, Asiatics now have their own class. They grow short scapes with long, distinctive "beaks" in northern climates but may not grow scapes at all in milder areas.

'Asian Tempest':
> A Korean garlic with large cloves. Taste is strong and hot raw, milder and fully developed when cooked. If harvested early it keeps nearly six months.

'Pyongyang' *(also called 'Pyong Vang')*:
> Crisp texture, hot flavor; rich and mild cooked. Stores well. Rich, reddish purple.

TURBAN

These are delicate-looking plants that sometimes send up a weak scape with a turban-shaped umbel. They're early, both to sprout in spring and to mature in summer, and they should be harvested after a couple of leaves have turned brown. Not known for long storage.

'Chinese Purple':
> Good in southern climates; ripens early yet is one of the longer-storing Turbans. Be careful of it raw—it's very hot.

'Thai Fire':
>Originated in Bangkok, brought to Salt Spring Island
in British Columbia by Dan Jason. It sprouts early,
sometimes while it's still in storage; typically bold,
hot taste.

CREOLE

Creoles originated in Spain, not Louisiana, although they grow well there; they also sometimes grow a scape. For a time they were lumped with Silverskins; then they were called Southern Continentals. Some people in the Southwest call them Mexican Purples, perhaps because they grow in lovely colors of red and purple. Because they have a sweet, rich taste, they're a good crop for a southern gardener with a yen to grow Rocamboles, which need a cold winter to grow a bulb. They're also long storing, which Rocamboles aren't. Gardeners in more northerly but not frigid regions have successfully grown Creoles, although they produce smaller bulbs in those areas.

'Burgundy':
>Sweet, rich, and mild, but never dull.
>A beautiful purple, squat bulb.

'Creole Red':
>A popular cultivar that arrived in California in
the 1980s. Has a fine, rich earthy flavor with just
enough bite. Stores seven or eight months.

'Morado de Pedronera':
>Came to the United States from Córdoba, Spain, in
1991. It has fat, full cloves and a hot, strong bite, unlike
most Creoles. Much mellower roasted or sautéed.

'Rose de Lautrec':
> The pride of Lautrec, France. A pink-skinned beauty
> with modest pungency. Warm, but not hot, faintly
> musky. Long storing.

Softneck

ARTICHOKE

This variety is often used commercially because it's easy to grow and produces large bulbs with many layers of cloves, the inner ones smaller than the outer layer. 'California Early' and 'California Late,' the varieties grown in Gilroy, California, the largest producer of fresh garlic in North America, are Artichokes. It's an adaptable plant that seldom bolts or grows a scape. Taste can be simple, without richness or depth, but many cultivars have good flavor.

'California Early':
> Flattish in shape, adaptable to many climates,
> early maturing; relatively mild, simple taste.

'California Late':
> Smaller and rounder bulbs than its sister garlic, with
> more cloves. Hotter in taste and longer storing than
> 'Early' and can bolt or form bulbils in the pseudostem
> in more northern climates.

'Inchelium Red':
> Voted the best-tasting garlic in a 1990 test done by
> *Organic Gardening* magazine. Interior cloves are a
> good size, unlike some other Porcelains. Pleasantly
> mild; produces less allicin than many varieties.

'Kettle River Giant':
>A flavorful Artichoke that stores well for six or
>seven months.

'Lorz Italian':
>Brought to Washington State in the 1800s by an
>Italian family. Good for mild winter areas but adapts
>to cooler climates, where it may partially bolt. Fine,
>complex flavor and stores well.

'Siciliano':
>Flavor is rich and zesty but not too hot; good raw and
>stores well.

SILVERSKIN

Silverskin is the variety usually sold in large quantities in super-markets because it stores well. Like Artichokes, Silverskins generally don't bolt, or grow a scape, though they will in climates with cold winters. They're also more apt than other varieties to produce a bulb the same year in the north if planted in early spring, probably because they don't need a period of vernalization. They're the latest garlics to mature and sometimes can be stored as long as a year, although long storage can make their hot, sulfurous taste stronger. The taste of cultivars varies, however, from mild to strong and acrid.

'Locati':
>Pinkish red, from Milan. Best sautéed lightly
>to temper the strong taste.

'Nootka Rose':
>From Waldron Island in Washington State.

The brownish cloves streaked with pink are very handsome. Many layers of cloves, with a rich, bold, medium-hot taste.

'Silver White':

It seems to grow anywhere, from maritime areas to places with warm or cold winters. Deceivingly mild at first, it explodes into intense heat that lasts. Lots of small inner cloves.

ACKNOWLEDGMENTS

*L*earning *about garlic* has taken me to many sources over many years, starting with the little Italian restaurant I stumbled into when I was seventeen. Its chef never realized what an impact his garlic-laden spaghetti and meatballs had on me, but I feel it necessary to thank him, wherever he is. I hope he's still happily cooking with garlic. I'm also grateful to other cooks of my youth who showed me how to use garlic in the kitchen, by example or just because they were daring enough—depending on their nationality—to use it.

After I started to grow garlic, thanks to the insistence of my friend Judith, the pace of my learning picked up. The speakers at the garlic fairs I attended provided me with bits of knowledge I scribbled in my notebook, and many books filled my brain with facts and fables about this unsung little vegetable, including its long history as a valuable medicine. On this note I especially want to thank Dr. Eric Block of the chemistry department at the University at Albany, State University of New York, author of the fascinating and informative *Garlic and Other Alliums: The Lore and the Science*, who gave me permission to refer to the material in his book, and I have done so liberally. Ted Jordan Meredith's *The Complete Book of Garlic: A Guide for Gardeners, Growers, and Serious Cooks*, was also a helpful resource. Longtime garlic lover and author Chester Aaron inspired me with his spirit and sent me his books to read. Paul Pospisil, editor of the *Garlic News*, which is an endless source of information in itself, answered my questions over the phone even while he was standing out in his garlic field.

I will be eternally grateful to Pauline Danigo in Lautrec, France, who translated for me on the day of the festival. Without her I would have been lost. My thanks also to Adrien Mucciante of Lautrec's tourist board, who made the village's history come alive for me; to Chrystel Pardessus of the Syndicat de Défense du Label Rouge, who explained the rules surrounding the growing of pink garlic; and to Dominique and Philippe Ducoudray, our gracious hosts at the enchanting Terrasse de Lautrec, who served delicious French breakfasts in their centuries-old garden, reputedly designed by the late, great André Le Nôtre.

Peter Ciccarelli, who handles media relations for the Gilroy Garlic Festival, saw that we had easy access to almost everything at the festival, and Larry Mickartz, owner and creative cook at Fitzgerald House bed and breakfast, generously acted as chauffeur on several occasions. Thanks again to you both.

Nancy Flight, associate publisher of Greystone Books, was a wonderful support during the writing of this book, asking for a little bit more here and a little less there in the most tactful terms. Barbara Czarnecki was a sensitive and intuitive copy editor on all fronts, but especially in helping to untangle the metric/imperial measurements and suggesting several stylish ways to circumvent them altogether.

Thanks also to my friends and family, who listened politely for a couple of years as I droned on about garlic's underestimated medicinal value, the politics of garlic (yes, they exist), and all the wonderful new cultivars available to us today. I apologize for becoming a garlic bore.

SOURCES

Below is a list of some of the places to buy garlic, to taste it, to celebrate it, and to read about it. It's far from exhaustive, but the Web, catalogs, and local media will yield more.

Garlic Festivals

UNITED STATES

EAT, DRINK, & STINK
Easton Garlic Fest
Easton, Pennsylvania
www.eastongarlicfest.com
Early October

GARLIC & HARVEST FESTIVAL
Bethlehem, Connecticut
www.garlicfestct.com
October, 2 days

GILROY GARLIC FESTIVAL
Gilroy, California
www.gilroygarlicfestival.com
Friday to Sunday,
Last Weekend of July

HUDSON VALLEY GARLIC FESTIVAL
Saugerties, New York
www.hudsonvalleygarlic.com
Late September, 2 days

MINNESOTA GARLIC FESTIVAL
Hutchinson, Minnesota
www.sfa-mn.org/garlicfest/
Mid-August, 1 day

NORTH QUABBIN GARLIC
& ARTS FESTIVAL
Orange, Massachusetts
www.garlicandarts.org
October, 2 days

NORTHWEST GARLIC FESTIVAL
Ocean Park, Washington
www.opwa.com
http://www.opwa.com/Ocean_Park_
Events/ocean_park_events.html
Late June, 2 days

SOUTHERN VERMONT
GARLIC & HERB FESTIVAL
Bennington, Vermont
www.lovegarlic.com
Early September, 2 days

CANADA
HILLS GARLIC FESTIVAL
New Denver, British Columbia
www.hillsgarlicfest.ca
Mid-September, 1 day

PERTH LIONS GARLIC FESTIVAL
Perth, Ontario
www.perthgarlicfestival.com
August, 2 days

STE-ANNE-DE-BELLEVUE
GARLIC FESTIVAL
Ste-Anne-de-Bellevue, Quebec
http://goingtoseed.wordpress.com
Late August, 1 day

SOUTH CARIBOO GARLIC FESTIVAL
Lac La Hache, British Columbia
www.garlicfestival.ca
Late August, 2 days

STINKING ROSE GARLIC FESTIVAL
Watershed Farm
Baker Settlement, Nova Scotia
camelia@pollinationproject.org
Late October, 1 day

STRATFORD GARLIC FESTIVAL
Stratford, Ontario
www.stratfordgarlicfestival.com
Mid-September, 2 days

FRANCE
FÊTE DE L'AIL ROSE
Lautrec, France
www.ailrosedelautrec.com
First Friday in August, 1 day

Where to Buy Garlic

UNITED STATES
BALDOR SPECIALTY FOODS
155 Food Center Drive
Bronx, New York 10474
718-860-9100
www.baldorfood.com
*Ail Rose de Lautrec and smoked
pink garlic, available in season only.*

CATSKILL MERINO SHEEP FARM
15½ Phillips Place
Goshen, New York 10924
wyatt@catskill-merino.com
www.catskill-merino.com
Organic garlic grown in
manure-enriched soil.

FILAREE FARM
182 Conconully Highway
Okanogan, Washington 98840
www.filareefarm.com
A major vendor of a wide
range of cultivars.

THE GARLIC STORE
5313 Mail Creek Lane
Fort Collins, Colorado 80525
thechiefclove@thegarlicstore.com
www.TheGarlicStore.com
Certified organic garlic.

GOURMET GARLIC GARDENS
Bangs, Texas 76823
www.gourmetgarlicgardens.com
Large website, growing and cooking
information, online farmers' market
with many varieties to order.

SWEDE LAKE FARMS
AND GLOBAL GARLIC
Watertown, Minnesota 55388
SwedeLakeFarms@yahoo.com
www.greatnorthernseedgarlic.com
Organic hardneck varieties.

CANADA
AUGUST'S HARVEST
4727 Road 130 RR #2
Gadshill, Ontario NOK 1J0
www.augustsharvest.com
info@augustsharvest.com
Certified organic garlic and shallots.

BEAVER POND ESTATES
3656 Bolingbroke Road
Maberly, Ontario KOH 2B0
garlic@rideau.net
Certified organic, 120 proven strains.

BOUNDARY GARLIC FARM
Box 273
Midway, British Columbia VOH 1MO
sonia@garlicfarm.ca
www.garlicfarm.ca
Large website, growing advice.
About fifty varieties for sale via mail
order; certified organic, heritage.

CLEAR SKY FARM
P.O. Box 19
Fort Steele, British Columbia
VOB 1NO
garlic@clearskyfarm.ca
www.clearskyfarm.ca
About a dozen organic hardneck
varieties. Also pickled scapes,
garlic chutney.

THE CUTTING VEG
25178 Valleyview Drive
Sutton West, Ontario LOE 1RO
www.thecuttingveg.com
daniel@thecuttingveg.com
*Organic, including Persian,
Tibetan, Ukrainian, Korean,
Italian, Yugoslavian, Sicilian.*

EUREKA GARLIC
RR #6
Kensington, Prince Edward
Island COB 1MO
al@eurekagarlic.ca
Many varieties, no chemicals.

MY FATHER'S GARLIC PATCH
1262 Cape Bear Road
Murray Harbour, Prince Edward
Island COA 1VO
myfathershouse@eastlink.ca
Organic garlic and veggies.

SALT SPRING SEEDS
Box 444, Ganges P.O.
Salt Spring Island, British
Columbia V8K 2W1
www.saltspringseeds.com
dan@saltspringseeds.com
*Dedicated to sustainable
agriculture. Large variety of garlic.*

Newsletter

Garlic News
3656 Bolingbroke Road
Maberly, Ontario KOH 2BO
garlic@rideau.net

Garlic Products and Gadgets

BLACK GARLIC INC.
www.blackgarlic.com

THE GARLIC MILL
AMPM Distribution
ZA Borio Novo
81570 Vielmur sur Agout
France
commandes@ampmdistribution.com
www.ampmdistribution.com

MICROPLANE RASPS
http://ca.microplane.com/
microplanekitchentools.aspx

LEE VALLEY TOOLS
www.leevalley.com

THE ULU FACTORY
211 West Ship Creek Avenue
Anchorage, Alaska 99501-1603
info@theulufactory.com
www.theulufactory.com

Recommended Reading

Aaron, Chester. *The Great Garlic
Book: A Guide with Recipes.*
Berkeley, CA: Ten Speed Press,
1997.
———. *Garlic Is Life: A Memoir with
Recipes.* Berkeley, CA: Ten Speed
Press, 1996.

Block, Eric. *Garlic and Other Alliums: The Lore and the Science*. Cambridge, UK: Royal Society of Chemistry, 2010.

Harris, Lloyd J. *The Book of Garlic, Revised Edition: New Recipes & Remedies, Folklore and Medical Data*. San Francisco, CA: Addison-Wesley, 1980.

——. *The Official Garlic Lovers Handbook*. San Francisco, CA: Aris Books, 1986.

Meredith, Ted Jordan. *The Complete Book of Garlic: A Guide for Gardeners, Growers, and Serious Cooks*. Portland, OR: Timber Press, 2008.

Renoux, Victoria. *For the Love of Garlic: The Complete Guide to Garlic Cuisine*. Garden City Park, NY: Square One Publishers, 2005.

Documentary

Blank, Les. *Garlic Is as Good as Ten Mothers*. El Cerrito, CA: Flower Films, 1980.

INDEX

RECIPE INDEX

almonds: Sopa de Ajo Blanco,
157–58
anchovy fillets: Salsa Verde, 163–64
Anna's Sauce, 44–45
avocado: Les Blank's Lunch, 165

bacon: Lentil, Bacon, and Tomato
Stew with Forty Cloves of Garlic,
160–61
basil: Anna's Sauce, 44–45
blueberries: Roasted Garlic,
Blueberry, and Pear Cobbler with
Garlic-Pecan Brickle Cream,
167–69
bread: Cold-Coming-On Soup, 158–
59; Les Blank's Lunch, 165; Sopa
de Ajo Blanco, 157–58

bread crumbs: Salsa Verde, 163–64
buttermilk: Roasted Garlic,
Blueberry, and Pear Cobbler with
Garlic-Pecan Brickle Cream,
167–69

capers: Salsa Verde, 163–64
cheese: Anna's Sauce, 44–45; Cold-
Coming-On Soup, 158–59;
Jacqueline Barthe's Creamy
Garlic Pie, 166–67; Whole-Hog
Potatoes, 165–66
chicken stock: Cold-Coming-On
Soup, 158–59; Lentil, Bacon, and
Tomato Stew with Forty Cloves
of Garlic, 160–61; Sopa de Ajo
Blanco, 157–58

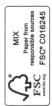